P9-DDB-731

THE SOUTH BEACH DIET
GOOD FATS GOOD CARBS GUIDE

Arthur Agatston, M.D.

Author of the *New York Times* Bestseller *The South Beach Diet*

RODALE

Notice

This book is intended as a reference volume only, not as a medical manual. The information given here is designed to help you make informed decisions about your health. It is not intended as a substitute for any treatment that may have been prescribed by your doctor. If you suspect that you have a medical problem, we urge you to seek competent medical help.

Mention of specific companies, organizations, or authorities in this book does not imply endorsement by the publisher, nor does mention of specific companies, organizations, or authorities imply that they endorse this book.

Internet addresses and telephone numbers given in this book were accurate at the time it went to press.

Sales of this book without a front cover may be unauthorized. If this book is coverless, it may have been reported to the publisher as "unsold or destroyed" and neither the author nor the publisher may have received payment for it.

© 2004 by Arthur Agatston, M.D.
All rights reserved. No part of this publication may be reproduced or transmitted in any form or by any means, electronic or mechanical, including photocopying, recording, or any other information storage and retrieval system, without the written permission of the publisher.

Special thanks to Kathleen Hanuschak, R.D., for her help in putting together all of the information in this guide.

Printed in the United States of America
Rodale Inc. makes every effort to use acid-free ∞, recycled paper ♻.

Book design by Carol Angstadt

ISBN: 1–57954–958–6

Distributed to the book trade by St. Martin's Press

4 6 8 10 9 7 5 3   paperback

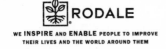

RODALE

WE **INSPIRE** AND **ENABLE** PEOPLE TO IMPROVE
THEIR LIVES AND THE WORLD AROUND THEM

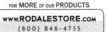

FOR MORE OF OUR PRODUCTS
WWW.RODALESTORE.COM
(800) 848-4735

CONTENTS

YOUR ROAD MAP
TO SOUTH BEACH SUCCESS

Welcome! I'm glad you've decided to try the South Beach Diet and have taken the first step toward a future filled with health and vitality.

The South Beach Diet can't be classified as a low-carb diet, a low-fat diet, or a high-protein diet. Its rules: Consume the right carbs and the right fats and learn to snack strategically. The South Beach Diet has been so widely successful because people lose weight without experiencing cravings or feeling deprived, or even feeling that they're *on* a diet. It allows you to enjoy "healthy" carbohydrates, rather than the kinds that contribute to weight gain, diabetes, and cardiovascular disease. You can eat a great variety of foods in a great variety of recipes. This prevents repetition and boredom, two obstacles to long-term success. Our goal is that the South

Beach Diet becomes a healthy lifestyle, not just a diet. The purpose of this guide is to help you to accomplish this with ease. Read on for more on the principles of the diet, how to use this Guide, and shopping and dining-out tips.

Good Fats, Bad Fats

Fat is an important part of a healthy diet. There's more and more evidence that many fats are good for us and actually reduce the risk of heart attack and stroke. They also help our sugar and insulin metabolism and therefore contribute to our goals of long-term weight loss and weight maintenance. And because good fats make foods taste better, they help us enjoy the journey to a healthier lifestyle. But not all fats are created equal—there are good fats and bad fats.

"Good" fats include monounsaturated fats, found in olive and canola oils, peanuts and other nuts, peanut butter, and avocados. Monounsaturated fats lower total and "bad" LDL cholesterol—which accumulates in and clogs artery walls—while maintaining levels of "good" HDL cholesterol, which carries cholesterol from artery walls and delivers it to the liver for disposal.

Omega-3 fatty acids—polyunsaturated fats found in coldwater fish, canola oil, flaxseeds, walnuts, almonds, and macadamia nuts—also count as good fat. Recent studies have shown that populations that eat more omega-3s, like Eskimos (whose diets are heavy on fish), have fewer serious health problems like heart disease and diabetes. There is evidence that omega-3 oils helps prevent or treat depression, arthritis, asthma, and colitis and help prevent cardiovascular deaths. You'll eat both monounsaturated fats and omega-3s in abundance in all three phases of the Diet.

"Bad fats" include saturated fats—the heart-clogging kind found in butter, fatty red meats, and full-fat dairy products.

"Very bad fats" are the manmade trans fats. Trans fats, which are created when hydrogen gas reacts with oil, are found in many packaged foods, including margarine, cookies, cakes, cake icings, doughnuts, and potato chips. Trans fats are worse than saturated fats; they are bad for our blood vessels, nervous systems, and waistlines.

As this Guide went to press, the Food and Drug Administration (FDA) ruled that by 2006, food manufacturers must list the amount of trans fats in their products on the label. (The natural trans fats in meat and milk, which act very differently in the body than the manmade kind, will not require labeling.) Until then, here are a few ways to reduce your intake of trans fats and saturated fats, South Beach style.

Go natural: Limit margarine, packaged foods, and fast food, which tend to contain high amounts of saturated and trans fats. **Make over your cooking methods:** Bake, broil, or grill rather than fry. **Lose the skin:** Remove the skin from chicken or turkey before you eat it. **Ditch the butter:** Cook with canola or olive oil instead of butter, margarine, or lard. **Slim down your dairy:** Switch from whole milk to fat-free or 1% milk.

Good Carbs, Bad Carbs

Carbohydrates, foods that contain simple sugars (short chains of sugar molecules) or starches (long chains of sugar

(continued on page 8)

The Trans-Fat Hot List

You've probably heard a lot in the news lately about trans fats—a particularly nasty type of fat that can wreak havoc on your health. Food manufacturers have not been required to list this type of fat on their food labels in the past, but because of new government regulations, manufacturers will be required to list the amount of trans fats in their products by 2006. Until then, here is what you need to know to identify trans fats present in foods.

Look for the words "hydrogenated" or "partially hydrogenated" oil on the list of ingredients. If it is listed as the first, second, or third ingredient, the food has a lot trans fats in it. The common names for trans fats to look for on food labels include partially hydrogenated soybean oil, partially hydrogenated corn oil, partially hydrogenated soybean and/or cottonseed oil, partially hydrogenated palm kernel oil, partially hydrogenated coconut oil, and partially hydrogenated vegetable oil shortening.

You can also refer to this "Hot List" of foods that are known to harbor trans fats. To keep your weight loss on track, and to maintain good health, it's best to avoid these foods as much as possible. There are plenty of great-tasting, healthier alternatives you can have instead—just check the food chart in this book!

BREADS AND BREAD PRODUCTS

Biscuits, made from mix

Biscuits or rolls, made from refrigerated dough

Coating mixes for fish, meat, or poultry

Stuffing mixes

Taco shells

White and wheat flour breads (some types)

BREAKFAST FOODS

Most commercial bakery items, such as:

Cinnamon buns

Danish

Doughnuts

Muffins

Pastries or bakery items with icing or frosting

Sweet rolls

Toaster tarts or strudel, plain or iced

CANDY

Most commercial confectionary, such as:

Caramels

Chocolate

Fruit chews

Hard candies with a creamy texture (some types)

Seasonal candy

Taffy-like candy

DESSERTS

Most commercially prepared items, such as:

Cake sprinkles, decorettes, or baking chips

Cakes and cake mixes

Cakes or cupcakes prepared with icing or frosting

Ice cream cakes

Pie crusts, such as traditional, graham cracker, and cookie crumb, and some pie fillings, such as chocolate

Pound cake and fat-free pound cake

Ready-to-spread frostings

(continued)

DESSERTS (CONT.)

Refrigerated cookie dough

Refrigerated cookie kits with icing

DIPS AND SNACKS

Bean dips (some types)

Cheese and pretzel snack kits

Cheese and cracker snack kits (some types)

Cheese puffs

Chocolate- or yogurt-covered snacks (most types)

Cookie snack kits

Cookies, most types such as chocolate chip and vanilla wafers

Corn chips

Crackers, including cheese-filled sandwich-type, cream-filled sandwich-type, saltine-type, snack crackers and some types of wheat crackers

Nacho cheese dips

Popcorn packaged for the microwave

Potato chips and potato sticks

Pretzels filled with imitation cheese

Pudding snacks, prepared

Tortilla chips (some types)

Weight-loss snack bars (some types)

FAST FOODS

Breakfasts with biscuit topping, made from biscuit mixes

Biscuits served with fast-food dinners

French fries

Fried apples or fast-food fruit pies

Fried chicken

Fried fish sandwiches

Mixed meals from a box that contain buttermilk biscuit topping, cornbread topping, dumplings, or pouched seasoning mix

Most deep-fried fast foods

FATS AND OILS

Light spreads (some types)

Margarine, hard stick and regular tub types

Vegetable shortening, regular and butter-flavored

FROZEN FOODS

Breaded fish sticks

Entrées (some types)

French fries

Fruit pies and pie crusts

Pancakes and French toast

Pastries, heat-and-eat or pastries with icing

Pizza and pizza crusts

Pot pies

Waffles and waffle sticks

MILK AND MILK PRODUCTS

International and instant latte coffees (some types)

Refrigerated fat-free nondairy creamers

Refrigerated nondairy creamers (some types)

Whipped toppings

SALADS AND SALAD DRESSINGS

Commercially prepared salad dressings (some types)

SOUPS AND STEWS

Bouillon cubes (some types)

Boxed onion soup and dip mix

Ramen noodle and soup cups (some types)

molecules), have been blamed for our epidemic of obesity and diabetes. This is only partially true, because there are both good and bad carbohydrates. The good carbs contain the important vitamins, minerals, and other nutrients that are essential to our health and that help prevent heart disease and cancer. The bad carbs, which have been consumed by Americans in unprecedented quantities (largely in an attempt to avoids fats), are the ones that have resulted in the fattening of America. Bad carbs are refined carbs, the ones where digestion has begun in factories instead of in our stomachs. The good carbs are the ones humans were designed to consume—the unrefined ones that have contributed to our health since we began eating! Unrefined carbohydrates are found in whole, natural foods, such as whole grains, legumes, rice, and starchy vegetables. They're also called complex carbohydrates, so named for their molecular structure. Besides being packed with fiber, vitamins, and minerals, good carbs take longer to digest—a good thing, as you'll soon see.

Refined carbohydrates, on the other hand, are found in packaged, processed foods, such as store-bought baked goods, crackers, pasta, and white bread.

Refined carbohydrates are made with white flour and contain little or no fiber. In fact, many products made with white flour are advertised as fortified with vitamins and minerals, because the process of turning grain into white flour strips away its fiber and nutrients. One of our South Beach Diet rules is to avoid foods labeled as "fortified." Current evidence is that fortification with vitamins does not recreate the benefits of the natural vitamins that have been removed.

Despite the fact that good carbs are a critical part of a healthy diet, the typical American diet is filled with the bad kinds. And when we're overweight as a result of a diet laden with bad carbs, our bodies' ability to process *all* carbohydrates goes awry. To understand why, you need to understand the role of the hormone insulin.

Insulin, Fat, and "Fast Sugar"

All foods, even natural foods like fruits and beans, contain naturally occurring sugar in some form. But there's a critical difference among these sugars: The body digests and absorbs them at different speeds.

When sugars from food enter the bloodstream, the pancreas produces insulin. It's insulin's job to move sugars out of the blood and into the cells, where they're either used or stored for future use. Insulin is the key that "unlocks" our cells and lets sugars in.

How much insulin is required to do that job depends on the foods we eat. Foods that are broken down and absorbed into the bloodstream quickly require a lot of insulin. Those that are metabolized and enter the blood more slowly require a gradual release of insulin.

In a nutshell, the quicker sugar floods the bloodstream, the quicker insulin rises. This is bad, both for your weight and for your general health.

Here's why: When glucose is absorbed slowly, the rise in

(continued on page 12)

Beyond Weight Loss: The South Beach Diet Benefits Your Health, Too

Has your doctor has told you that you must lose weight to stave off heart disease or diabetes? Then the South Beach Diet may be the one for you.

Why? Because the Diet that's helping millions across the nation shed their extra pounds *didn't start out as a weight-loss diet at all*. I created the Diet to help my patients lower their levels of cholesterol and triglycerides and to lower their risk of pre-diabetes (the condition that precedes full-blown type 2 diabetes and that has been linked to risk of heart attack and stroke).

And it's been proven to do just that.

To give just one example, one of my male patients in his midfifties had high blood pressure, high cholesterol, high triglycerides, and narrowing in his coronary arteries. His previous doctor had prescribed the usual medications. But once on the Diet, his cardiac profile quickly improved. His triglycerides, which had been over 400, fell below 100—a normal level—after just a month. He also lost 30 pounds, which he's kept off, and no longer takes all those heart medications.

The results of the Diet have also been measured in a scientific setting. My colleagues and I conducted a study pitting the Diet against the strict "step 2" American Heart Association diet. They randomized 40 overweight volunteers to either of the diets, meaning that half went on the Heart Association program and half got the South Beach Diet. None of the subjects knew where their diet had come from.

After 12 weeks, five patients on the Heart Association diet had given up, compared with one on the South Beach plan. The South Beach patients also showed a greater decrease in waist-to-hip ratio, suggesting a true decrease in cardiac risk. Triglycerides dramatically decreased for the South Beach dieters, and their good-to-bad cholesterol ratio improved more than that of the Heart Association group. Finally, the South Beach dieters experienced a mean weight loss of 13.6 pounds, almost double the 7.5 pounds lost by the Heart Association group.

blood sugar is gradual—and so is its fall, once insulin begins to work. A slow decline in blood sugar means fewer cravings later.

But when blood sugar rises quickly, the pancreas pumps out a correspondingly high level of insulin. The result? Blood sugar drops so low that it triggers new cravings. Often, we satisfy cravings by overeating (typically bad carbs like chips and candy bars), which leads to weight gain. Worse, the excess weight caused by overeating can lead to insulin resistance, the precursor to full-blown type 2 diabetes. In insulin resistance, cells ignore insulin's signal to accept glucose from the blood. As a result, the pancreas must crank out huge amounts of insulin until eventually the exhausted organ wears out.

Those of us who have grown protruding bellies while our arms and legs stay relatively thin are likely to have the syndrome of insulin resistance or "pre-diabetes." This occurs commonly in people with a family history of diabetes. Another sign of this syndrome is the occurrence of fatigue, weakness, headaches, irritability, shakiness, and cravings in the late morning or late afternoon. These are signs of exaggerated falls in blood sugar levels. The consumption of refined carbohydrates has unmasked this syndrome in approximately 25 percent of Americans and in the great majority of those of us who are overweight.

While eating the South Beach way will result in weight loss, it will also correct the way your body reacts to the very foods that made you heavy. It increases your body's sensitivity to insulin, thereby decreasing the swings in blood sugar that cause us to be hungry again, too soon after we finish a meal.

This metabolic transformation occurs in three phases. The purpose of Phase 1 is to eradicate your cravings. You will accomplish this by eliminating all starches including all breads, potatoes, and rice. You will also eliminate all sugars, including all fruits and alcoholic beverages. You will enjoy strategic snacking, eating healthy snacks like nuts or low-fat cheese before your blood sugar dips too low in the late morning afternoon and/or evening. It takes much fewer calories to prevent those afternoon cravings than it does to satisfy those cravings once they hit. In Phase 1, nutrient rich vegetables and healthy salads are encouraged. You can expect to lose between 7 and 13 pounds during Phase 1.

In Phase 2, you'll gradually add back good carbohydrates, such as whole fruits and whole grains. Here's the principle for adding more carbs back safely: Do it gradually and attentively. The goal is to eat more carbs again while continuing to lose weight. If you add an apple and a slice of bread a day and you're still dropping pounds, that's great. If you try having an apple, two slices of bread, and a banana daily and notice that your weight loss has stalled, you've gone too far. It's time to cut back, or try some different carbs and monitor the results. You can enjoy a glass of red or white wine with a meal; drinking wine with a meal actually helps slow digestion. In this phase, weight loss is about 1 to 2 pounds per week. You learn which carbs you can enjoy without the return of cravings.

Once you have reached your weight loss goal, it is time for Phase 3, the maintenance phase. There are no absolute restrictions here, but you have learned the "pecking order" of the important food groups. You have learned to choose brown rice instead of white rice, sweet potatoes instead of white potatoes, and pita bread rather than white bread. This is where the South Beach Diet becomes a lifestyle. (For an idea of which foods to avoid and which foods to enjoy on the South Beach Diet, see the lists on the next pages.)

In the next section, you'll be introduced to a system that can help you limit foods that cause unhealthy, fat-producing spikes and dips in blood sugar and insulin and choose those that keep blood sugar steady, making it easier to lose weight and keep it off.

Introducing the Glycemic Index

The glycemic index (GI) is a system that ranks foods by how fast and how high they cause blood sugar to rise after eating a particular food. The GI of any particular food is always compared to a standard reference food, which is either one slice of white bread or a small amount of glucose, both of which have a numerical value of 100. The higher the glycemic index, the greater the swings in blood sugar produced. So, in general, the lower the glycemic index, the better the food choice. For mixed meals, the total glycemic index is approximately the average of the indices of the individual foods.

Generally speaking, you can think of GI in 3 ranges: "low" (55 and below), "medium" (56 to 69), and "high" (70 or above).

Foods with a low GI are converted to glucose more slowly, and so their sugars enter the bloodstream more slowly.

Foods with a medium or high GI, which are converted to glucose more quickly, release their sugars into the bloodstream more rapidly. This results in a swifter rise in insulin.

Unrefined carbs often fall lower on the GI scale because they're rich in fiber, which takes longer to digest and so results in a slow, gradual rise in blood sugar.

How about refined, bad carbs? Not surprisingly, their processed sugars enter the bloodstream quickly. This quick conversion makes blood sugar and insulin rise and fall quickly—definitely not so good.

On the South Beach Diet, you'll tend to eat foods that fall lower on the GI, prepared or eaten in ways that allow your body to digest and absorb them more slowly. After Phase 1, the strictest phase of the Diet, you'll reintroduce good carbohydrates with a higher GI.

While the GI is an astounding breakthrough in our understanding of how carbohydrates affect our metabolism, there are a few important things you need to know to use the system successfully. First, the GI doesn't account for portion size. The solution: the concept of the glycemic load (GL), which takes into account a food's GI (the quality of carbohydrate) as well as the amount (the quantity of carbohydrate) per serving. It also represents the load, or stress, placed on the pancreas from the amount of carbohydrates consumed from a particular food or meal.

For this Guide, our evaluation of each food choice is based on the glycemic index, glycemic load, and on other factors as well. We don't include a dedicated column with a GI number for each entry because that information is not

(continued on page 22)

15

Phase 1

The following is a list of foods that you can feel free to enjoy (as well as foods you'll need to avoid) when you begin Phase 1 of the South Beach Diet. These lists will help you stay on track and avoid carbohydrates that may crop up in foods where you don't expect them.

Foods to Enjoy

BEEF
Lean cuts, such as:
Sirloin (including ground)
Tenderloin
Top round

DAIRY
1% or fat-free milk
Plain fat-free yogurt
Low-fat plain soy milk (4 g of fat or less per serving)
1% or fat-free buttermilk

POULTRY (SKINLESS)
Cornish hen
Turkey bacon (2 slices per day)
Turkey and chicken breast

SEAFOOD
All types of fish and shellfish

PORK
Boiled ham
Canadian bacon
Tenderloin

VEAL
Chop
Cutlet, leg
Top round

LUNCHMEAT
Fat-free or low-fat only

CHEESE (REDUCED FAT)
American
Cheddar
Cottage cheese, 1%, 2%, or fat-free
Cream cheese substitute, dairy-free

Feta
Mozzarella
Parmesan
Provolone
Ricotta
String

NUTS
Almonds, 15
Cashews, 15
Macadamias, 8
Peanut butter, 2 tbsps
Peanuts, 20 small
Pistachios, 30

EGGS
Whole eggs are not limited
unless otherwise directed by
your doctor. Use egg whites
and egg substitute as desired.

TOFU
Use soft, low-fat, or lite
varieties

**VEGETABLES AND
LEGUMES**
Artichokes
Asparagus
Beans
Broccoli
Cabbage

Cauliflower
Celery
Collard greens
Cucumbers
Eggplant
Lettuce (all varieties)
Mushrooms (all varieties)
Snow peas
Spinach
Sprouts, alfalfa
Tomatoes
Turnips
Water chestnuts
Zucchini

FATS
Oil, canola
Oil, olive

SPICES AND SEASONINGS
All spices that contain no
added sugar
Broth
Extracts (almond, vanilla, or
others)
Horseradish sauce
I Can't Believe It's Not Butter!
spray
Pepper (black, cayenne, red,
white)

(continued)

Foods to Enjoy (cont.)

SWEET TREATS (LIMIT TO 75 CALORIES PER DAY)

Candies, hard, sugar-free

Chocolate powder, no sugar added

Cocoa powder, baking type

Fudge pops, no sugar added

Gelatin, sugar-free

Gum, sugar-free

Popsicles, sugar-free

Sugar substitute

Foods to Avoid

BEEF
Brisket

Liver

Other fatty cuts

Rib steaks

POULTRY
Chicken, wings and legs

Duck

Goose

Poultry products, processed

PORK
Honey-baked ham

VEAL
Breast

CHEESE
Brie

Edam

Non reduced-fat

VEGETABLES

Beets

Corn

Potatoes, sweet

Potatoes, white

Yams

FRUIT

Avoid all fruits and fruit juices in Phase 1, including:

Apples

Apricots

Berries

Cantaloupe

Grapefruit

Peaches

Pears

STARCHES AND CARBS

Avoid all starchy food in Phase 1, including:

Bread, all types

Cereal

Matzo

Oatmeal

Pasta, all types

Pastry and baked goods, all types

Rice, all types

DAIRY

Avoid the following dairy in Phase 1:

Ice cream

Milk, whole or 2%

Soy milk

Yogurt, cup-style and frozen

MISCELLANEOUS

Alcohol of any kind, including beer and wine

Phase 2

As with Phase 1, Phase 2 also has recommendations for which foods to eat. The first list tells you which foods to reintroduce into your diet. The second list includes foods that you'd best eat only rarely—any more than that could affect your blood glucose levels and derail your weight-loss efforts as well.

Foods You Can Reintroduce to Your Diet

VEGETABLES/LEGUMES
Barley
Beans, pinto
Black-eyed peas
Carrots

STARCHES (LIMIT)
Bagels, small, whole grain
Bread
  multigrain
  oat and bran
  rye
  whole wheat
Cereal
  Fiber One
  Kellogg's Extra-Fiber All-Bran
  oatmeal (not instant)
  other high-fiber
  Uncle Sam

Muffins, bran, sugar-free (no raisins)
Pasta, whole wheat
Peas, green
Pita
  stone-ground
  whole wheat
Popcorn
Potato, small, sweet
Rice
  brown
  wild

FRUIT
Apples
Apricots, dried or fresh
Blueberries
Cantaloupe
Cherries

Grapefruit
Grapes
Kiwi
Mangoes
Oranges
Peaches
Pears
Plums
Strawberries

DAIRY

Artifically sweetened nonfat flavored yogurt, 4 oz cup per day

MISCELLANEOUS

Chocolate (sparingly)
  bittersweet
  semisweet
Pudding, fat-free, sugar-free
Wine, red or white

Foods to Avoid or Eat Rarely

VEGETABLES
Beets
Corn
Potatoes

STARCHES AND BREADS
Bagel, refined wheat
Bread
  refined wheat
  white
Cookies
Cornflakes
Matzo
Pasta, white flour
Potatoes
  baked, white
  instant

Rice cakes
Rice, white
Rolls, dinner

FRUIT
Bananas
Canned fruit, juice-packed
Fruit juice
Pineapple
Raisins
Watermelon

MISCELLANEOUS
Honey
Ice cream
Jam

available for all of the 1,200 foods that are listed in these pages.

Our recommendations are meant to be guidelines, not absolute do's and don'ts. As we learn more, there will certainly be changes in future editions.

A good diet is always a work in progress, because scientists are always conducting new and better research. In reading this guide, you will notice that our recommendations on a few key foods have changed since the original South Beach Diet book was published. Specifically, we now allow you to eat as many tomatoes as you want, even in Phase 1. Though technically a fruit, tomatoes have a low GI number and contain a lot of nutrients. Carrots, too, have gone from being banned to being allowed in Phase 2, due to new research on their glycemic index value. Finally, and for many of you most importantly, our recommendation on dairy has changed. Although milk contains some lactose sugars, recent studies have shown that lactose may help control body fat. You can't consume whole milk, which is high in saturated fat, but you can enjoy 1% or fat-free milk or plain fat-free yogurt in Phase 1. To keep abreast of all changes and new recommendations for the diet, visit www.southbeachdiet.com/updates regularly.

HOW TO USE
THE FOOD GUIDE

The South Beach Diet doesn't require you to count calories or fat or carbohydrate grams. But bad carbs and bad fats have a way of sneaking up on you, especially when you're dining out or eating on the run. This Guide gives you the knowledge you need to make healthy food choices. Use it faithfully, and you'll be virtually guaranteed to stick to South Beach principles—anytime, anywhere.

The more than 1,200 foods in this Guide are listed in alphabetical order by category. Each entry lists the total amount of carbohydrates, sugar, and fat for one portion. In the last column is our recommendation for how to incorporate this food into your diet. This recommendation is based on many factors including the glycemic index, the glycemic load, the fiber and nutrient content of the food, and more. Within specific categories, the recommendation assigned to each food is usually either "Good," "Limited," "Very Limited," or "Avoid." In a few instances, we use "Allowed," for foods where implying quantities might be misleading. Sugar substitutes are one example of that. But it's possible that the foods you are buying in your supermarket are different than what we've analyzed for this guide, even if it's the same *type* of food. So remember to read the labels! Watch out for canned foods thickened with cornstarch or other starches, powdered mixes that contain trans fats, and sugar additives like high-fructose corn syrup.

These recommendations are guidelines, not hard and fast quantifiers, because so much depends on you as an individual. How often you might eat something depends on which Phase of the diet you are on, how much weight you're trying to lose, your body's own metabolism, and so on. The best way to use this guide is to first consult the allowable foods list for whatever Phase you're on, and refer to any specific eating recommendations. Certain categories of foods like whole fruits are identified as "good" because they are in fact good, healthy foods, but if you're in Phase 1 of the diet you still need to avoid them entirely. When you do reintroduce more good carbs in Phase 2 and beyond, do so with discretion and pay attention to how your body responds. The South Beach Diet is not just a way of eating; it's a way of thinking about food. Once you understand its principles, you'll always be able to make the right food choices.

BEANS AND LEGUMES

Beans and legumes are excellent sources of soluble fiber, which delays stomach emptying time, slows glucose absorption, and can lower blood cholesterol and assist weight loss. Beans are also an excellent source of protein for vegetarians. Soy protein, found in soybeans and soybean products, lowers LDL (bad) cholesterol. We recommend liberal consumption of these healthy foods.

Avoid canned beans that contain brown sugar, lard, or molasses.

BEANS

Food	Portion	Total Carbs (g)	Total Sugar (g)	Total Fat (g)	Recmmd.
Aduki beans, boiled	½ cup	19	2	0	Good
Baked beans					
Homemade, w/sugar	½ cup	27	11	5	Very Limited
Plain, vegetarian, canned	½ cup	26	8	0	Good
W/bacon and brown sugar, canned	½ cup	30	13	3	Avoid
W/beef, canned	½ cup	22	6	5	Limited
W/honey and mustard, canned	½ cup	31	12	0	Avoid
W/pork, canned	½ cup	25	8	2	Limited
Black beans, canned	½ cup	17	1	1	Good
Black-eyed peas, frozen	½ cup	20	3	1	Good
Black turtle soup beans, presoaked, boiled	½ cup	21	4	0	Good

BEANS (CONT.)

Food	Portion	Total Carbs (g)	Total Sugar (g)	Total Fat (g)	Recmmd.
Butter beans, canned	½ cup	18	1	0	Good
Calico beans, cooked	½ cup	24	2	0	Good
Chickpeas, canned, drained	½ cup	22	1	2	Good
Chickpeas (hummus)	½ cup	24	2	5	Good
Chili, vegetarian, canned	½ cup	19	3	0	Good
Chili, w/turkey and beans, canned	½ cup	13	3	1	Good
Chili con carne, w/beans, canned	½ cup	16	2	5	Good
Chili con carne, w/meat, canned	½ cup	8	1	12	Avoid
Kidney beans, red, canned, or boiled	½ cup	19	2	0	Good
Kidney beans, white, boiled	½ cup	21	2	1	Good
Lentils, brown, boiled	½ cup	20	2	0	Good
Lentils, pink or red, boiled	½ cup	24	2	0	Good
Lima beans, frozen, reheated	½ cup	17	2	0	Good
Mung beans, cooked	½ cup	19	2	0	Good

Food	Portion	Total Carbs (g)	Total Sugar (g)	Total Fat (g)	Recmmd.
Navy beans, pressure-cooked	½ cup	24	2	1	Good
Pinto beans, canned	½ cup	18	1	1	Good
Refried beans					
Fat-free, canned	½ cup	18	1	0	Good
Prepared w/corn oil	½ cup	20	1	5	Limited
Prepared w/lard, nonhydrogenated	½ cup	23	1	6	Avoid

PEAS

Food	Portion	Total Carbs (g)	Total Sugar (g)	Total Fat (g)	Recmmd.
Green peas, canned, drained	½ cup	16	4	0	Good
Green sugar snap peas, fresh or frozen	½ cup	7	3	0	Good
Snow peas, pod, raw	½ cup	5	3	0	Good
Split peas, boiled	½ cup	21	3	0	Good

SOYBEANS

Food	Portion	Total Carbs (g)	Total Sugar (g)	Total Fat (g)	Recmmd.
Black soybeans, canned	½ cup	9	1	2	Good
Green soybeans (edamame) frozen	½ cup	7	2	4	Good

SOYBEANS (CONT.)

Food	Portion	Total Carbs (g)	Total Sugar (g)	Total Fat (g)	Recmmd.
Yellow fermented soybeans (natto)	½ cup	13	3	10	Good
Yellow soybeans, boiled	½ cup	9	3	8	Good

SPROUTS, BEAN

Food	Portion	Total Carbs (g)	Total Sugar (g)	Total Fat (g)	Recmmd.
Kidney bean sprouts, raw	½ cup	4	1	0	Good
Lentil sprouts, raw	½ cup	9	1	0	Good
Mung bean sprouts, raw	½ cup	3	1	0	Good

BEVERAGES

Most carbonated beverages are pure sugar and a source of empty calories. Diet sodas are okay in moderation, but water is the best choice for quenching thirst and hydrating your body. Both coffee and tea are major contributors of caffeine to our diets. Too much caffeine can cause a drop in blood sugar, leading to hunger and cravings. Flavored coffees and mixes can be a source of hidden sugars. Commercial fruit juices are frequently concentrates of the fruit's sugar without any of the fiber. You get much more nutritional benefit out of eating a whole fruit. If you need your glass of OJ in the morning, fresh squeezed is best.

Finally, research suggests that moderate consumption of alcohol reduces risk for heart disease and diabetes. We believe this is best accomplished by drinking red or white wine with meals. Beer is the worst choice because it contains maltose, the sugar with the highest glycemic index. All alcohol is off-limits in Phase 1.

BEVERAGES, ALCOHOLIC

Food	Portion	Total Carbs (g)	Total Sugar (g)	Total Fat (g)	Recmmd.
Beers					
Lager	12 fl oz	6	0	0	Avoid
Light	12 fl oz	4	4	0	Avoid
Regular	12 fl oz	11	10	0	Avoid
Liquors (gin, rum, vodka, whiskey)	1½ fl oz	0	0	0	Very Limited
Mixed drinks					
Rum and coke	1 standard recipe drink	26	26	0	Avoid
Vodka and orange juice from frozen concentrate	1 standard recipe drink	30	29	0	Avoid
Vodka and tomato juice	1 standard recipe drink	9	7	0	Very Limited
Wines, cooking					
Marsala	2 Tbsp	3	3	0	Avoid
Red/white	2 Tbsp	1	1	0	Avoid
Sherry	2 Tbsp	2	2	0	Avoid
Wines, dessert					
Madeira	2 fl oz	5	5	0	Avoid
Port	2 fl oz	5	5	0	Avoid
Sherry	2 fl oz	5	5	0	Avoid
Wines, table					
Burgundy	5 fl oz	2	2	0	Good
Claret	5 fl oz	2	2	0	Good
Red	5 fl oz	3	3	0	Good

BEVERAGES, ALCOHOLIC (CONT.)

Food	Portion	Total Carbs (g)	Total Sugar (g)	Total Fat (g)	Recmmd.
Wines, table (cont.)					
Rose	5 fl oz	2	2	0	Good
White	5 fl oz	1	1	0	Good
Wine spritzer	12 fl oz	3	3	0	Good

BEVERAGES, NONALCOHOLIC

Food	Portion	Total Carbs (g)	Total Sugar (g)	Total Fat (g)	Recmmd.
Carbonated drinks					
Club soda	12 fl oz	0	0	0	Allowed
Cola	12 fl oz	39	39	0	Avoid
Cream soda	12 fl oz	42	42	0	Avoid
Ginger ale	12 fl oz	32	32	0	Avoid
Ginseng-type soda	12 fl oz	39	39	0	Avoid
Grape soda	12 fl oz	42	42	0	Avoid
Lemon-lime soda	12 fl oz	38	38	0	Avoid
Orange soda	12 fl oz	48	48	0	Avoid
Pepper-type soda	12 fl oz	38	38	0	Avoid
Root beer	12 fl oz	38	38	0	Avoid
Seltzer water	12 fl oz	0	0	0	Allowed
Soda, diet, artificially sweetened	12 fl oz	0	0	0	Limited

Food	Portion	Total Carbs (g)	Total Sugar (g)	Total Fat (g)	Recmmd.
Sparkling mineral water	12 fl oz	0	0	0	Good
Coffee, brewed					
Black, regular	8 fl oz	0	0	0	Limited
Black, decaf	8 fl oz	0	0	0	Allowed
Coffee, cappuccino and espresso					
Cappuccino, prepared, w/milk and sugar	8 fl oz	10	10	4	Avoid
Espresso	1 fl oz	0	0	0	Limited
Coffee, instant					
Coffee substitute, cereal grain, prepared, black	8 fl oz	0	0	0	Allowed
Flavored, international-type, sugar-free, prepared from mix	8 fl oz	5	0	0	Limited
Flavored, international-type, w/sugar, prepared from mix	8 fl oz	10	8	1	Avoid

BEVERAGES, NONALCOHOLIC (CONT.)

Food	Portion	Total Carbs (g)	Total Sugar (g)	Total Fat (g)	Recmmd.
Dairy drinks and mixes					
Carob-flavored drink, prepared w/milk, from mix	8 fl oz	23	14	8	Avoid
Chocolate flavored drink, prepared w/milk, from mix	8 fl oz	31	30	9	Avoid
Hot chocolate/ cocoa, prepared w/milk, from mix	8 fl oz	29	22	6	Avoid
Milkshake, chocolate	12 fl oz	62	60	13	Avoid
Milkshake, strawberry	12 fl oz	64	63	10	Avoid
Milkshake, vanilla	12 fl oz	61	60	10	Avoid
Strawberry instant drink, prepared w/milk, from mix	8 fl oz	33	32	8	Avoid
Strawberry instant drink, prepared w/water, from mix	8 fl oz	26	25	0	Avoid

Food	Portion	Total Carbs (g)	Total Sugar (g)	Total Fat (g)	Recmmd.
Juice-flavored drinks, sweetened					
Cranberry-apple or grape	8 fl oz	42	42	0	Avoid
Cranberry juice cocktail	8 fl oz	36	36	0	Avoid
Fruit punch, pouch-type	8 fl oz	30	30	0	Avoid
Lemonade, homemade	8 fl oz	26	23	0	Avoid
Orange juice drink, prepared w/water, from instant drink mix	8 fl oz	23	23	0	Avoid
Pouch-type, prepared	8 fl oz	30	30	0	Avoid
Sports drink, Gatorade-type, w/glucose, ready to drink	8 fl oz	15	15	0	Avoid
Soy milk shake, vanilla	12 fl oz	36	32	9	Avoid
Soy smoothie drink, banana	12 fl oz	36	30	4	Avoid
Teas					
Brewed tea, black	8 fl oz	0	0	0	Allowed

BEVERAGES, NONALCOHOLIC (CONT.)

Food	Portion	Total Carbs (g)	Total Sugar (g)	Total Fat (g)	Recmmd.
Teas (cont.)					
Brewed tea, black, w/1 tsp sugar	8 fl oz	4	4	0	Very Limited
Brewed tea, herbal	8 fl oz	0	0	0	Allowed
Iced tea, instant, sweetened w/sugar, prepared w/water, from mix	8 fl oz	17	17	0	Avoid
Iced tea, ready to drink, sweetened w/high fructose corn syrup, bottled	8 fl oz	17	17	0	Avoid
Iced tea, unsweetened/ diet iced tea	8 fl oz	0	0	0	Allowed

BREAD AND BREAD PRODUCTS

Like grains, bread and bread products can be enjoyed often if you eat the right ones. Whole grain breads are the best choice. Whole grain products should read "100 percent whole wheat," "whole oats," or "whole rye." Watch out for breads that are labeled "whole wheat" rather than "whole grain." While some nutrients may be preserved, the glycemic index is generally just as high as that of white bread. Look for at least 3 grams of fiber per serving. Other good choices are pita, whole grain pumpernickel, and sourdough bread. But remember, according to the guidelines for Phase 2, you do have to moderate your consumption of breads and starches once they are reintroduced to your diet.

Anything labeled "fortified" means that processing has removed essential vitamins and nutrients. Any attempts to return vitamins artificially are unlikely to be sufficient. Avoid "fortified" foods and commercial breads that include hydrogenated oils.

BREAD

Food	Portion	Total Carbs (g)	Total Sugar (g)	Total Fat (g)	Recmmd.
Bagels					
Blueberry	3 oz	40	10	1	Avoid
Cinnamon raisin	3 oz	47	2	1	Avoid
Egg	3 oz	45	1	2	Avoid
Plain, onion, or sesame	3 oz	45	1	1	Avoid
Poppy seed	3 oz	49	1	1	Avoid
Whole wheat	3 oz	48	2	1	Avoid
Bread					
Baguette, white, plain	1 oz	21	0	1	Avoid
Baguette, w/1 tsp butter	1 oz	21	0	6	Avoid

Food	Portion	Total Carbs (g)	Total Sugar (g)	Total Fat (g)	Recmmd.
Bread (cont.)					
Barley, prepared w/flour and 50% barley kernels	1 oz	19	1	1	Limited
Barley, prepared w/100% flour	1 oz	16	1	1	Limited
Buckwheat	1 oz	14	1	1	Limited
Cinnamon raisin	1 oz	14	4	1	Avoid
Cornbread, prepared from baking mix	3 oz	30	4	6	Avoid
Cracked wheat, coarse	1 oz	14	1	1	Limited
Focaccia	2 oz	23	2	4	Avoid
French	1 oz	15	0	1	Avoid
Gluten-free, wheat-free	1 oz	13	1	1	Very Limited
High protein	1 oz	12	1	0	Limited
Honey oat	1 oz	14	2	1	Very Limited
Italian	1 oz	14	1	1	Avoid
Multigrain, 7-grain bread	1 oz	14	1	1	Limited
Oat bran	1 oz	11	1	1	Limited
Pita pocket, wheat, unleavened, 6"	1 each	35	1	2	Limited

Food	Portion	Total Carbs (g)	Total Sugar (g)	Total Fat (g)	Recmmd.
Pita pocket, white, unleavened, 6"	1 each	33	1	1	Limited
Potato	1 oz	14	1	1	Avoid
Pumpernickel, whole grain	1 oz	13	1	1	Limited
Rice, high amylose	1 oz	12	0	1	Limited
Rice, low amylose	1 oz	12	0	1	Avoid
Rye, light	1 oz	14	2	1	Limited
Rye, w/linseed	1 oz	15	2	1	Limited
Sourdough bread, rye	1 oz	15	0	1	Limited
Soy and flaxseed	1 oz	12	2	1	Limited
Sprouted wheat	1 oz	13	1	1	Limited
Stone-ground whole wheat bread	1 oz	14	1	1	Limited
Vienna	1 oz	15	0	1	Avoid
White, enriched	1 oz	14	1	1	Avoid
Whole wheat, made w/enriched wheat flour	1 oz	13	1	1	Avoid

BREAD PRODUCTS

Food	Portion	Total Carbs (g)	Total Sugar (g)	Total Fat (g)	Recmmd.
Bread crumbs					
Dry, plain	1 oz	21	1	2	Avoid

BREAD PRODUCTS (CONT.)

Food	Portion	Total Carbs (g)	Total Sugar (g)	Total Fat (g)	Recmmd.
Bread crumbs (cont.)					
Gluten-free, wheat-free	1 oz	14	1	3	Avoid
Soft, white	1 oz	15	1	1	Avoid
Breadsticks, plain	1 oz	20	1	1	Avoid
Bread stuffing, prepared	½ cup	43	3	9	Avoid
Croutons, plain, dry	1 oz	21	1	2	Avoid
Rolls					
Frankfurter/hot dog roll	1½ oz	19	3	2	Very Limited
Hamburger bun	1½ oz	22	5	3	Very Limited
Hoagie roll	4¾ oz	68	5	5	Avoid
Kaiser	2 oz	30	3	2	Avoid
Potato	2 oz	24	4	4	Avoid
Sourdough rye	2 oz	30	1	1	Limited
Whole grain	2 oz	30	1	1	Limited
Taco shell, baked	1 each	9	0	3	Avoid
Tortilla, corn, unleavened, soft, 6"	1 each	12	0	1	Very Limited
Tortilla, wheat flour, unleavened, soft, 6"	1 each	18	0	2	Limited

BREAKFAST FOODS

Man was designed to consume much more fiber than we get in modern diets. Fiber slows our digestion and thereby helps prevent swings in our sugar and insulin levels. Both hot and cold breakfast cereals can be excellent sources of fiber; choose ones with a fiber content in the 6 gram or higher range. Hot oatmeal cereals are excellent but only those that are slow cooked; instant hot cereals have too high glycemic indices. And don't be fooled by cereals labeled "natural." Many types, including granola, have plenty of sugar and minimal fiber. Even worse, they may have hydrogenated oils.

Donuts are the worst breakfast choice. They have high levels of trans fats and highly processed flour with a very high glycemic index. Avoid store-bought muffins as well, because they are usually loaded with sugars.

BREAKFAST BARS

Food	Portion	Total Carbs (g)	Total Sugar (g)	Total Fat (g)	Recmmd.
Granola bar, almond nut	1¾ oz	30	14	12	Avoid
Granola bar, oatmeal raisin	1½ oz	28	23	6	Avoid
Kudos Bar–type, whole grain, chocolate chip	1⅓ oz	25	16	6	Avoid
Sports bar, Power Bar–type, chocolate	2¼ oz	45	14	2	Avoid

CEREALS, COLD, DRY

Food	Portion	Total Carbs (g)	Total Sugar (g)	Total Fat (g)	Recmmd.
All-Bran	1 oz (½ cup)	22	5	1	Good
All-Bran, extra fiber	1 oz (½ cup)	21	0	1	Good

CEREALS, COLD, DRY (CONT.)

Food	Portion	Total Carbs (g)	Total Sugar (g)	Total Fat (g)	Recmmd.
Bran Buds	1 oz (⅓ cup)	23	8	1	Limited
Bran Chex	1 oz (½ cup)	23	5	1	Limited
Bran Flakes	1 oz (¾ cup)	23	5	1	Limited
Cheerios	1 oz (1 cup)	23	6	1	Limited
Corn Chex	1 oz (1 cup)	24	3	0	Avoid
Corn Flakes	1 oz (1 cup)	24	2	0	Avoid
Corn Pops	1 oz (1 cup)	26	12	0	Avoid
Crispix	1 oz (1 cup)	24	3	0	Avoid
Fruit Loops	1 oz (1 cup)	25	13	1	Avoid
Frosted Flakes	1 oz (¾ cup)	26	12	0	Avoid
Golden Grahams	1 oz (¾ cup)	24	10	1	Avoid
Granola, homemade w/old-fashioned oats, honey, and almonds	1 oz (¼ cup)	19	6	5	Very Limited
Grape Nuts	1 oz (¼ cup)	23	3	1	Avoid
Life	1 oz (¾ cup)	22	6	1	Limited
Muesli, Swiss	1 oz (¼ cup)	22	7	2	Limited
Nutri-Grain	1 oz (¾ cup)	24	4	0	Limited
Puffed rice	1 oz (2 cups)	25	0	0	Avoid
Puffed wheat	1 oz (2 cups)	22	0	0	Avoid
Raisin Bran	1 oz (½ cup)	22	9	1	Very Limited
Rice Chex	1 oz (1¼ cup)	25	2	0	Avoid
Rice Krispies	1 oz (1¼ cup)	25	2	0	Avoid

Food	Portion	Total Carbs (g)	Total Sugar (g)	Total Fat (g)	Recmmd.
Shredded wheat	1 oz (2 biscuits)	24	0	0	Limited
Special K	1 oz (1 cup)	21	3	0	Limited
Team	1 oz (1 cup)	24	11	1	Avoid
Total	1 oz (1⅓ cup)	23	4	0	Avoid

CEREALS, HOT, COOKED, PREPARED WITH WATER

Food	Portion	Total Carbs (g)	Total Sugar (g)	Total Fat (g)	Recmmd.
Buckwheat groats	½ cup	17	1	1	Good
Cream of Rice, instant	½ cup	14	0	0	Avoid
Cream of Wheat	½ cup	14	0	0	Limited
Cream of Wheat, instant	½ cup	16	1	1	Avoid
Farina	½ cup	12	1	0	Avoid
Maypo	½ cup	16	4	1	Limited
Millet	½ cup	21	0	1	Avoid
Oat bran	½ cup	13	0	1	Good
Oatmeal					
Instant	½ cup	12	0	1	Avoid
Old-fashioned	½ cup	12	0	1	Good
Quick	½ cup	26	2	3	Limited

CEREALS, TOPPINGS

Food	Portion	Total Carbs (g)	Total Sugar (g)	Total Fat (g)	Recmmd.
Almonds	6 pieces	1	0	4	Good

CEREALS, TOPPINGS (CONT.)

Food	Portion	Total Carbs (g)	Total Sugar (g)	Total Fat (g)	Recmmd.
Flaxseed, ground	1 Tbsp	3	0	3	Good
Honey, pure	1 tsp	17	17	0	Very Limited
Lecithin granules	1 Tbsp	1	0	5	Limited
Oat bran, unprocessed	2 Tbsp	8	0	0	Good
Psyllium husks	1 Tbsp	1	0	0	Good
Raisins	2 Tbsp	14	12	0	Very Limited
Rice bran, crude	2 Tbsp	7	0	3	Good
Sugar	1 tsp	4	4	0	Very Limited
Wheat bran, unprocessed	2 Tbsp	4	0	0	Good
Wheat germ	1 Tbsp	3	1	1	Good

FAST FOOD BREAKFAST SANDWICHES

Food	Portion	Total Carbs (g)	Total Sugar (g)	Total Fat (g)	Recmmd.
Biscuit w/bacon and egg	1 each	29	3	31	Avoid
Biscuit w/bacon, egg, and cheese	1 each	33	3	31	Avoid
Croissant					
W/bacon, egg, and cheese	1 each	24	3	28	Avoid
W/ham, egg, and cheese	1 each	24	3	34	Avoid

Food	Portion	Total Carbs (g)	Total Sugar (g)	Total Fat (g)	Recmmd.
W/sausage, egg, and cheese	1 each	25	3	38	Avoid
English muffin w/egg, cheese, and Canadian bacon	1 each	29	3	13	Avoid

PANCAKES AND WAFFLES

Food	Portion	Total Carbs (g)	Total Sugar (g)	Total Fat (g)	Recmmd.
Pancakes					
Buckwheat, plain, prepared from gluten-free batter mix, 5"	1 each	20	3	4	Limited
Buttermilk, plain, prepared from batter mix, 5"	1 each	21	5	6	Avoid
Potato, homemade, 4"	1 each	19	2	6	Avoid
Whole wheat, prepared from batter mix, 5"	1 each	18	4	5	Very Limited
Waffles					
Belgian, frozen	1 each	30	7	6	Avoid
Blueberry, frozen, 4"	1 each	15	4	3	Avoid
Buttermilk, frozen, 4"	1 each	15	1	3	Avoid

PASTRIES

Food	Portion	Total Carbs (g)	Total Sugar (g)	Total Fat (g)	Recmmd.
Apple bun, fat-free	3 oz	43	22	0	Avoid
Croissant, cheese, medium	3 oz	27	2	12	Avoid
Doughnuts					
Chocolate	2 oz	29	15	14	Avoid
Chocolate, w/chocolate icing	2½ oz	36	21	14	Avoid
Crème-filled, Bavarian	2½ oz	33	12	11	Avoid
Crème-filled, Boston	2¾ oz	38	17	11	Avoid
Cruller, glazed	3 oz	45	28	14	Avoid
Cruller, powdered sugar	2½ oz	35	11	15	Avoid
Éclair, chocolate, w/custard	3 oz	42	21	12	Avoid
Glazed, mini, Munchkin-type	1 each	10	7	3	Avoid
Jelly-filled	2½ oz	33	17	10	Avoid
Plain, w/chocolate icing	2½ oz	30	15	14	Avoid
Plain, w/vanilla icing	2½ oz	32	13	10	Avoid
Honey bun, glazed or iced	2 oz	47	22	17	Avoid
Jelly-filled sweet roll	3 oz	45	20	13	Avoid

Food	Portion	Total Carbs (g)	Total Sugar (g)	Total Fat (g)	Recmmd.
Muffins					
Blueberry	2 oz	27	6	4	Avoid
Bran	2 oz	28	5	4	Avoid
Carrot	2 oz	24	8	3	Avoid
Chocolate chip	2 oz	27	8	7	Avoid
Fat-free	2 oz	25	14	0	Avoid
Lemon poppy seed	2 oz	22	11	5	Avoid
Muffins, English					
Cinnamon raisin	1 each	27	2	2	Avoid
Plain	1 each	26	2	1	Very Limited
Whole wheat	1 each	30	2	1	Limited
Scone, fat-free	2 oz	15	4	0	Very Limited
Scone, regular	2 oz	25	6	9	Avoid
Sticky bun, cinnamon raisin	3 oz	43	20	14	Avoid
Toaster pastry					
Fruit-filled	1 each	37	17	5	Avoid
Fruit-filled w/frosting	1 each	37	20	5	Avoid
Strudel, w/fruit	1 each	26	10	9	Avoid

CANDY AND CANDY BARS

Most candy is pure sugar and as such should be avoided.

However, if you are going to indulge, a small quantity of dark chocolate is the best choice. The only negative about chocolate is its sugar content, and dark chocolate has a lower sugar content than other types.

There are now many varieties of low–carb, sugar-free, or diabetic candies on the market. Many use sugar alcohols such as sorbitol or mannitol as sweeteners. These sugar alcohols are sweet tasting, but instead of being absorbed into the bloodstream, they remain in the intestines. Consuming candy with these sugar alcohols can cause some stomach upset and diarrhea.

Food	Portion	Total Carbs (g)	Total Sugar (g)	Total Fat (g)	Recmmd.
Almonds, carob-coated	1 oz	13	7	10	Very Limited
Almonds, milk chocolate–coated	1 oz	13	6	11	Very Limited
Candy corn	1 oz	26	26	0	Avoid
Chocolate candy bar					
Plain	1½ oz	25	19	14	Avoid
W/almonds	1½ oz	22	18	14	Avoid
W/nougat filling	2 oz	34	28	14	Avoid
Fruit candy, Skittles-type	1 oz	26	22	1	Avoid
Fudge, chocolate walnut	1 oz	21	19	5	Avoid
Fudge, peanut butter	1 oz	16	15	5	Avoid
Gum, sugar-free, w/sorbitol	1 stick	4	0	0	Limited

Food	Portion	Total Carbs (g)	Total Sugar (g)	Total Fat (g)	Recmmd.
Gumdrops	1 oz	28	25	0	Avoid
Gummy Bears	1 oz	28	25	0	Avoid
Hard candy, Life Savers–type, peppermint	1 oz	28	18	0	Avoid
Hard candy, sugar-free, artificially sweetened	1 oz	25	0	0	Limited
Jelly beans	1 oz	27	17	0	Avoid
Marshmallows, regular-size	2 pieces	13	10	0	Avoid
Milk chocolate candy kisses	1 oz	17	14	9	Avoid
Peanut brittle, homemade	1 oz	20	19	5	Avoid
Peanuts, chocolate-covered, w/candy coating	1 oz	17	14	7	Very Limited
Raisins, chocolate-covered	1 oz	20	17	5	Avoid
Soy nuts, chocolate-covered	1 oz	15	12	10	Very Limited

CHEESE, CHEESE PRODUCTS, AND CHEESE SUBSTITUTES

Whole milk cheeses are a source of saturated fat, so choose low-fat or fat-free cheese for most of your eating and snacking. Mozzarella cheese sticks make particularly convenient and healthy snacks. Occasionally, however, it's okay to enjoy a small amount of a very flavorful cheese such as blue cheese or Parmesan occasionally, because a little goes a long way to enhance the flavor of a dish without contributing a substantial amount of saturated fat.

CHEESE

Food	Portion	Total Carbs (g)	Total Sugar (g)	Total Fat (g)	Recmmd.
Asiago	1 oz	1	1	8	Limited
Blue	1 oz	1	1	8	Limited
Brie	1 oz	0	0	8	Avoid
Camembert	1 oz	0	0	7	Avoid
Cheddar					
Fat-free	1 oz	1	0	0	Good
Low-fat	1 oz	1	0	2	Good
Reduced-fat	1 oz	1	0	5	Limited
Regular	1 oz	0	0	9	Avoid
Colby	1 oz	1	1	9	Avoid
Cottage cheese					
Creamed, 4% milk fat	½ cup	3	1	5	Avoid
Fat-free	½ cup	6	5	0	Good
Low-fat, 1% milk fat	½ cup	3	3	1	Good
Reduced-fat, 2% milk fat	½ cup	4	4	2	Limited

Food	Portion	Total Carbs (g)	Total Sugar (g)	Total Fat (g)	Recmmd.
Cream cheese					
Fat-free	2 Tbsp	3	1	0	Good
Light, low-fat	2 Tbsp	2	2	5	Good
Regular	2 Tbsp	1	1	10	Avoid
Regular, whipped	3 Tbsp	1	1	11	Avoid
Edam	1 oz	0	0	8	Avoid
Feta	1 oz	1	1	6	Limited
Feta, reduced-fat	1 oz	1	1	3	Good
Fontina	1 oz	0	0	8	Avoid
Goat cheese, hard	1 oz	1	1	10	Avoid
Goat cheese, soft	1 oz	0	0	6	Limited
Gorgonzola	1 oz	0	0	9	Avoid
Gouda	1 oz	1	1	8	Avoid
Gruyère	1 oz	0	0	9	Avoid
Havarti	1 oz	1	1	8	Avoid
Jarlsberg	1 oz	1	1	8	Avoid
Limburger	1 oz	0	0	8	Avoid
Mascarpone	1 oz	1	1	13	Avoid
Monterey Jack					
Fat-free	1 oz	1	1	0	Good
Reduced-fat	1 oz	1	0	6	Limited
Regular	1 oz	0	0	9	Avoid

CHEESE (CONT.)

Food	Portion	Total Carbs (g)	Total Sugar (g)	Total Fat (g)	Recmmd.
Mozzarella					
Fat-free	1 oz	1	1	0	Good
Part skim	1 oz	1	1	5	Good
Whole milk	1 oz	1	0	6	Limited
Muenster	1 oz	0	0	9	Avoid
Neufchâtel	1 oz	1	1	6	Limited
Parmesan	1 oz	1	1	8	Limited
Parmesan/ Romano, grated	1 Tbsp	0	0	2	Good
Provolone, reduced-fat	1 oz	1	0	5	Good
Provolone, regular	1 oz	1	1	8	Limited
Ricotta, part skim	½ cup	6	2	10	Good
Ricotta, whole milk	½ cup	4	2	16	Avoid
Roquefort	1 oz	1	1	9	Limited
String cheese	1 oz	1	1	5	Limited
Swiss					
Fat-free	1 oz	3	1	0	Good
Reduced-fat	1 oz	1	1	6	Limited
Regular	1 oz	1	1	8	Avoid
Yogurt cheese, low-fat	1 oz	2	2	0	Good

CHEESE PRODUCTS

Food	Portion	Total Carbs (g)	Total Sugar (g)	Total Fat (g)	Recmmd.
American cheese, processed, prewrapped	1 oz	2	1	6	Limited
Cheddar cheese, extra sharp, cheese food	1 oz	3	2	7	Avoid
Cheez Whiz–type cheese sauce					
Light	2 Tbsp	6	6	3	Avoid
Regular	2 Tbsp	2	2	7	Avoid
Squeezable	2 Tbsp	4	4	8	Avoid
Jalapeño cheese, processed	1 oz	2	1	7	Avoid
Pimiento cheese, processed	1 oz	2	1	6	Avoid

CHEESE SUBSTITUTES (DAIRY-FREE)

Food	Portion	Total Carbs (g)	Total Sugar (g)	Total Fat (g)	Recmmd.
Rice Cheddar cheese	1 oz	5	0	3	Good
Soy cheese	1 oz	1	0	5	Good
Soy cream cheese	1 oz	1	0	8	Limited

CONDIMENTS

Some condiments can contain added sweeteners such as sugar, honey, corn syrup, and/or high-fructose corn syrup. Be sure to read the list of ingredients before you purchase.

Food	Portion	Total Carbs (g)	Total Sugar (g)	Total Fat (g)	Recmmd.
Chili sauce, sweetened	1 Tbsp	5	4	0	Avoid
Cocktail sauce, sweetened	1 Tbsp	4	4	0	Avoid
Horseradish	1 tsp	0	0	0	Good
Ketchup, sweetened	1 Tbsp	4	4	0	Avoid
Lemon juice	1 Tbsp	0	0	0	Good
Lime juice	1 Tbsp	0	0	0	Good
Mustard	1 tsp	0	0	0	Good
Salsa, homemade, w/oil	2 Tbsp	5	3	3	Limited
Salsa, ready-to-serve, no oil	2 Tbsp	4	2	0	Good
Soy sauce	1 Tbsp	2	2	0	Limited
Steak sauce	1 Tbsp	2	2	0	Avoid
Tabasco sauce	1 Tbsp	0	0	0	Good
Taco sauce	1 Tbsp	2	2	0	Limited
Tartar sauce	1 Tbsp	2	1	4	Avoid
Teriyaki sauce	1 Tbsp	3	1	0	Very Limited
Vinegar	2 Tbsp	1	1	0	Good
Worcestershire sauce	1 tsp	1	0	0	Good

CRACKERS, DIPS, AND SNACKS

Most crackers and packaged snack foods contain trans fats and should be avoided.

CRACKERS

Food	Portion	Total Carbs (g)	Total Sugar (g)	Total Fat (g)	Recmmd.
Animal crackers	1 oz	21	12	4	Avoid
Butter crackers, round-type	1 oz	17	1	7	Avoid
Cheese crackers	1 oz	16	1	8	Avoid
Crispbread, rye	1 oz	23	1	0	Avoid
Graham crackers	1 oz	22	5	3	Avoid
Matzoh	1 oz	24	1	0	Avoid
Melba toast	1 oz	22	1	1	Avoid
100% Stoned wheat crackers	1 oz	19	0	5	Limited
Oyster crackers	1 oz	20	0	3	Avoid
Saltines	1 oz	20	0	3	Avoid
Sandwich crackers, w/cheese filling	1 package	19	4	13	Avoid
Sandwich crackers, w/peanut butter filling	1 package	22	5	9	Avoid
Soda crackers	1 oz	20	0	3	Avoid
Water crackers	1 oz	23	0	3	Avoid

DIPS

Food	Portion	Total Carbs (g)	Total Sugar (g)	Total Fat (g)	Recmmd.
Bacon and horseradish	2 Tbsp	3	1	5	Avoid

DIPS (CONT.)

Food	Portion	Total Carbs (g)	Total Sugar (g)	Total Fat (g)	Recmmd.
Black bean	2 Tbsp	5	1	0	Good
Blue cheese, reduced-fat	2 Tbsp	4	2	7	Avoid
Chili and cheese	2 Tbsp	3	1	3	Limited
Clam	2 Tbsp	3	1	4	Limited
Eggplant (baba ghannoush)	2 Tbsp	2	1	6	Good
Guacamole, avocado	2 Tbsp	4	1	4	Good
Hummus	2 Tbsp	5	1	1	Good
Nacho cheese	2 Tbsp	2	1	5	Avoid
Ranch, reduced-fat	2 Tbsp	5	1	8	Avoid
Sour cream and onion	2 Tbsp	2	1	5	Avoid

SNACKS

Food	Portion	Total Carbs (g)	Total Sugar (g)	Total Fat (g)	Recmmd.
Bagel chips	1 oz	21	1	3	Avoid
Banana chips, sweetened	1 oz	17	11	10	Avoid
Beef jerky	1 oz	1	1	7	Avoid
Caramel apple	1 medium apple	51	45	5	Avoid
Cheese puffs or cheese curls	1 oz	15	1	10	Avoid
Chex party mix, traditional	1 oz	21	3	4	Avoid

Food	Portion	Total Carbs (g)	Total Sugar (g)	Total Fat (g)	Recmmd.
Corn chips	1 oz	16	0	9	Avoid
Cracker Jack, plain	1 oz	23	15	2	Avoid
Fruit Roll-Ups– type, dried fruit snack	1 oz	15	5	1	Avoid
Popcorn					
Air-popped, plain	2 cups	12	0	0	Limited
Air-popped, w/1 tsp butter	2 cups	12	0	5	Avoid
Air-popped, w/1 tsp oil	2 cups	12	0	5	Limited
Cheese popcorn	2 cups	12	0	7	Avoid
Microwave popcorn, plain	2 cups	12	0	0	Avoid
Potato chips					
Fat-free	1 oz	18	0	0	Avoid
Plain	1 oz	15	0	10	Avoid
Potato sticks	1 oz	15	0	10	Avoid
Reduced-fat	1 oz	19	0	6	Avoid
Pretzels					
Fat-free	1 oz	22	1	0	Avoid
Hard, baked	1 oz	22	1	2	Avoid
Low-fat	1 oz	23	1	1	Avoid
Soft pretzel, w/mustard	3 oz	45	2	1	Avoid
Whole wheat	1 oz	23	0	1	Avoid

SNACKS (CONT.)

Food	Portion	Total Carbs (g)	Total Sugar (g)	Total Fat (g)	Recmmd.
Rice cakes					
Flavored	1 each	12	4	1	Avoid
Oriental mix	1 each	15	3	7	Avoid
Plain	1 each	8	0	0	Very Limited
Tortilla chips	1 oz	18	0	7	Avoid
Trail mix, traditional, w/raisins and nuts	1 oz	17	14	11	Avoid

DESSERTS

Desserts are fairly limited on the initial phase of the South Beach Diet, although you can feel free to enjoy sugar-free gelatin or one of our healthy and satisfying ricotta cheese combinations. Fruits, particularly berries, are ideal Phase 2 desserts. Strawberries dipped in dark chocolate are a personal favorite! Remember, the darker the chocolate, the lower the sugar content.

Many food manufacturers began adding partially hydrogenated fats—trans fats—to replace the previously used saturated fats in commercial goods as a way of preserving their shelf lives. Trans fats are common in cookies and baking mixes. Trans fats are worse than saturated fats and should be avoided as much as possible.

CAKES

Food	Portion	Total Carbs (g)	Total Sugar (g)	Total Fat (g)	Recmmd.
Angel food cake	2 oz	29	23	0	Avoid
Banana bread	2 oz	30	19	7	Avoid
Boston cream pie (sponge cake w/custard, no glaze)	3 oz	39	25	8	Avoid

Food	Portion	Total Carbs (g)	Total Sugar (g)	Total Fat (g)	Recmmd.
Cake, plain, average, unfrosted	1 oz	15	8	5	Avoid
Cheesecake, chocolate	2¾ oz	33	25	21	Avoid
Cheesecake, plain	2¾ oz	22	19	20	Avoid
Chocolate cake, from packet mix, w/chocolate frosting	2¾ oz	42	38	13	Avoid
Chocolate cake, from packet mix, w/vanilla frosting	2¾ oz	40	30	13	Avoid
Coffee cake, w/nuts	2 oz	29	18	15	Avoid
Pound cake, made w/butter	2 oz	28	16	11	Avoid
Sponge cake, plain	2 oz	23	16	1	Very Limited
Vanilla layer cake, Pepperidge Farm–type	2¾ oz	43	23	13	Avoid
Yellow cake, from packet mix, w/chocolate frosting	2¾ oz	37	24	11	Avoid
Yellow cake, from packet mix, w/vanilla frosting	2¾ oz	38	29	10	Avoid

COOKIES

Food	Portion	Total Carbs (g)	Total Sugar (g)	Total Fat (g)	Recmmd.
Arrowroot biscuit	3 small biscuits (½ oz)	12	6	3	Avoid
Butter cookie	2 cookies (1 oz)	21	9	6	Avoid
Fig bar	1 bar (½ oz)	11	7	1	Avoid
Gingersnap	3 small cookies (¾ oz)	16	7	3	Avoid
Oatmeal	1 cookie (⅔ oz)	10	5	3	Avoid
Peanut butter, homemade	1 cookie (¾ oz)	12	7	5	Avoid
Sandwich cookie					
Chocolate crème-filled	2 cookies (¾ oz)	15	8	4	Avoid
Peanut butter crème-filled	2 cookies (1 oz)	18	8	6	Avoid
Vanilla crème-filled	2 cookies (¾ oz)	15	8	4	Avoid
Shortbread	2 cookies (1 oz)	19	10	7	Avoid
Tea biscuit	2 biscuits (⅔ oz)	15	8	2	Avoid
Vanilla wafer	7 small wafers (1 oz)	21	10	4	Avoid

GELATIN

Food	Portion	Total Carbs (g)	Total Sugar (g)	Total Fat (g)	Recmmd.
Sugar-free, prepared	½ cup	0	0	0	Good

Food	Portion	Total Carbs (g)	Total Sugar (g)	Total Fat (g)	Recmmd.
W/fruit, prepared	½ cup	25	25	0	Avoid
W/sugar, prepared	½ cup	19	19	0	Avoid

PIES

Food	Portion	Total Carbs (g)	Total Sugar (g)	Total Fat (g)	Recmmd.
Apple fruit pie, two crusts	⅙ of 8" pie (4 oz)	43	21	12	Avoid
Blueberry fruit pie, two crusts	⅙ of 8" pie (4 oz)	41	17	11	Avoid
Cherry crumb pie	⅙ of 8" pie (4 oz)	50	30	15	Avoid
Chocolate chiffon pie	⅛ of 8" pie (4 oz)	41	17	15	Avoid
Chocolate peanut butter pie	⅛ of 8" pie (4 oz)	37	15	15	Avoid
Peach fruit pie, two crusts	⅙ of 8" pie (4 oz)	45	31	12	Avoid
Pumpkin pie	⅛ of 8" pie (4 oz)	30	17	10	Avoid

PUDDING AND MOUSSE

Food	Portion	Total Carbs (g)	Total Sugar (g)	Total Fat (g)	Recmmd.
Pudding					
Bread pudding, homemade, w/cinnamon raisin bread	⅓ cup	21	15	5	Avoid

PUDDING AND MOUSSE (CONT.)

Food	Portion	Total Carbs (g)	Total Sugar (g)	Total Fat (g)	Recmmd.
Pudding (cont.)					
Egg custard, homemade, or no-bake recipe, prepared	½ cup	16	16	7	Avoid
Instant, prepared w/reduced-fat milk, chocolate	½ cup	28	21	2	Avoid
Instant, prepared w/reduced-fat milk, vanilla	½ cup	30	19	2	Avoid
Rice pudding, homemade, prepared w/whole milk and long-grain rice	½ cup	30	19	4	Avoid
Tapioca pudding	½ cup	28	22	4	Avoid
Mousse					
Butterscotch, reduced-fat, prepared from mix	½ cup	10	1	3	Avoid
Chocolate, reduced-fat, prepared from mix	½ cup	10	1	3	Avoid
Mixed berry, reduced-fat, prepared from mix	½ cup	9	1	3	Avoid

Food	Portion	Total Carbs (g)	Total Sugar (g)	Total Fat (g)	Recmmd.
Vanilla, reduced-fat, prepared from mix	½ cup	8	1	3	Avoid

EGGS, EGG DISHES, AND EGG SUBSTITUTES

The good news is that eggs are okay. It is true that eggs are high in cholesterol, but they are also low in saturated fat. Eggs are rich in protein and the yolk is a good source of natural vitamin E. Eggs do increase cholesterol minimally, but they also increase HDL, the good cholesterol. Omelets are a great way of including lots of healthful vegetables in your breakfast, while hard-boiled eggs have the advantage of being fast and convenient. If you don't like the yolk, egg white omelets made from Egg Beaters are good choices. So if you love eggs, go ahead and enjoy!

EGGS, FRESH

Food	Portion	Total Carbs (g)	Total Sugar (g)	Total Fat (g)	Recmmd.
Extra large	1 each	0	0	5	Good
Large	1 each	0	0	5	Good
Medium	1 each	0	0	4	Good
Small	1 each	0	0	4	Good
White only	1 extra-large	0	0	0	Good
Yolk only	1 extra-large	0	0	5	Good

EGGS, OTHER

Food	Portion	Total Carbs (g)	Total Sugar (g)	Total Fat (g)	Recmmd.
Duck	1 large	0	0	10	Avoid
Goose	1 large	0	0	19	Avoid

EGGS, OTHER (CONT.)

Food	Portion	Total Carbs (g)	Total Sugar (g)	Total Fat (g)	Recmmd.
Omega-3 fat enriched	1 large	0	0	5	Good
Quail	3 each	0	0	3	Good
Turkey	1 large	0	0	10	Avoid

EGG DISHES

Food	Portion	Total Carbs (g)	Total Sugar (g)	Total Fat (g)	Recmmd.
Boiled, 1 large	1 serving	0	0	5	Good
Deviled, 2 halves	1 serving	1	0	10	Good
Fried, 1 large egg w/1 tsp butter	1 serving	0	0	10	Limited
Fried, 1 large egg w/1 tsp trans-free margarine	1 serving	0	0	10	Good
Omelets, 2-egg					
Plain, w/1 tsp butter	1 serving	1	1	14	Limited
Plain, w/1 tsp trans-free margarine	1 serving	1	1	13	Good
W/1 oz regular cheese	1 serving	2	0	29	Limited
W/1 oz regular cheese + 1 oz ham	1 serving	2	0	32	Limited
Extras: vegetables	½ cup	5	0	0	Good

Food	Portion	Total Carbs (g)	Total Sugar (g)	Total Fat (g)	Recmmd.
Omelets, 3-egg					
Plain, w/2 tsp butter	1 serving	1	1	22	Limited
Plain, w/2 tsp trans-free margarine	1 serving	1	1	21	Good
W/2 oz regular cheese	1 serving	3	0	48	Limited
W/2 oz regular cheese + 2 oz ham	1 serving	3	0	52	Limited
Omelets w/egg substitutes					
½ cup egg substitute w/1 tsp butter	1 serving	2	0	9	Limited
½ cup egg substitute w/1 tsp trans-free margarine	1 serving	1	1	7	Limited
Extras: ham	1 oz	0	0	2	Good
Extras: reduced-fat cheese	1 oz	1	0	5	Good
Extras: vegetables	½ cup	5	0	0	Good
Pickled, 1 large egg	1 serving	0	0	5	Good
Poached, 1 large egg	1 serving	0	0	5	Good

EGG DISHES (CONT.)

Food	Portion	Total Carbs (g)	Total Sugar (g)	Total Fat (g)	Recmmd.
Scrambled					
1 large egg, w/1 Tbsp fat-free milk + 1 tsp butter	1 serving	1	1	8	Limited
1 large egg, w/1 Tbsp fat-free milk + 1 tsp trans-free margarine	1 serving	1	1	8	Good
2 large eggs, w/2 Tbsp fat-free milk + 2 tsp butter	1 serving	2	1	18	Limited
2 large eggs, w/2 Tbsp fat-free milk + 2 tsps trans-free margarine	1 serving	2	1	16	Good

EGG SUBSTITUTES

Food	Portion	Total Carbs (g)	Total Sugar (g)	Total Fat (g)	Recmmd.
Liquid	¼ cup	1	1	2	Good
Powdered	⅓ oz	2	2	1	Good

FAST FOOD

Most fast foods fall into the "avoid" category. They are dripping with saturated fats, trans fats, sugars, and empty calories. But there are ways to eat wisely, even at a fast-food restaurant: Choose broiled or grilled food over deep-fried foods, and choose burgers without all the toppings and special sauces. Look for the salad bar. When you go out for pizza, choose thin-crust vegetarian pizzas. The tomato sauce may play a role in preventing prostate cancer due to lycopene, an antioxidant found in tomato products.

FAST FOOD BURGERS, SANDWICHES, AND WRAPS

Food	Portion	Total Carbs (g)	Total Sugar (g)	Total Fat (g)	Recmmd.
Bacon and cheese quesadilla	1 each	33	1	21	Avoid
BLT soft taco	1 each	21	3	22	Avoid
Burrito, w/beef	1 each	47	2	16	Avoid
Cheeseburger					
Double, w/condiments, on a bun	1 each	38	9	30	Avoid
W/bacon, on a bun	1 each	35	10	36	Avoid
W/condiments, on a bun	1 each	36	7	16	Avoid
Chicken fajita wrap	1 each	51	3	20	Avoid
Fish sandwich, breaded, on a bun, w/tartar sauce	1 each	45	5	23	Avoid
Grilled chicken BBQ sandwich	1 each	43	9	13	Avoid
Grilled chicken sandwich, w/mayonnaise	1 each	32	5	10	Very Limited
Hamburger, w/condiments, on a bun	1 each	35	7	10	Very Limited
Hot dog, on a bun					
Plain	1 each	19	4	12	Avoid

65

FAST FOOD BURGERS, SANDWICHES, AND WRAPS (CONT.)

Food	Portion	Total Carbs (g)	Total Sugar (g)	Total Fat (g)	Recmmd.
Hot dog, on a bun (cont.)					
W/chili and cheese	1 each	27	4	21	Avoid
W/chili and sauce	1 each	31	7	14	Avoid
Nachos, w/cheese	1 each	34	2	18	Avoid
Roast beef sandwich, on a bun, w/horseradish	1 each	35	7	14	Avoid

FAST FOOD CHICKEN

Food	Portion	Total Carbs (g)	Total Sugar (g)	Total Fat (g)	Recmmd.
Breast, crispy	1 piece (5 oz)	16	0	25	Avoid
Breast, extra crispy	1 piece (6 oz)	17	0	28	Avoid
Chicken nuggets	4-piece serving	13	0	11	Avoid
Chicken nuggets	6-piece serving	20	0	17	Avoid
Chicken nuggets	9-piece serving	29	0	25	Avoid
Drumstick, crispy	1 piece (2 oz)	4	0	9	Avoid
Drumstick, extra crispy	1 piece (2½ oz)	7	0	12	Avoid
Popcorn chicken	3½-oz serving	21	0	23	Avoid

Food	Portion	Total Carbs (g)	Total Sugar (g)	Total Fat (g)	Recmmd.
Thigh, crispy	1 piece (3½ oz)	6	0	18	Avoid
Thigh, extra crispy	1 piece (4 oz)	14	0	27	Avoid
Wings, honey BBQ	6-pieces (5 oz)	33	18	38	Avoid
Wings, hot	6 pieces (5 oz)	18	0	33	Avoid

FAST FOOD POTATO ITEMS

Food	Portion	Total Carbs (g)	Total Sugar (g)	Total Fat (g)	Recmmd.
Baked potato, large russet, w/skin, plain	10 oz potato	71	5	0	Avoid
Baked potato, large russet, w/skin, w/sour cream	10 oz potato	73	5	5	Avoid
French fries					
Large order	1 each	68	5	26	Avoid
Medium order	1 each	57	3	22	Avoid
Small order	1 each	26	2	10	Avoid
Mashed potatoes w/gravy	5 oz serving	17	5	6	Avoid

FATS AND OILS

With all the bad press fat has gotten over the last couple of decades, most Americans have concluded that just limiting fats makes a diet healthy. This was a major mistake. While limiting saturated fat (meat- and dairy-derived) and avoiding trans fats (manmade hydrogenated and partially hydrogenated oils) as completely as possible is important, the Mediterranean oils, including olive oil and omega-3 fish oils, appear to be good for both our blood vessels and our waistlines. There is no advantage to low-fat diet dressings that substitute sugars and starches for healthful oils. Along with a healthy oil, the vinegar in vinaigrette and oil-and-vinegar dressings is acidic and helps slow digestion. This lowers the glycemic index of the whole meal. Remember that nuts are also excellent sources of good fats and have been shown to help prevent heart attacks and strokes.

FATS

Food	Portion	Total Carbs (g)	Total Sugar (g)	Total Fat (g)	Recmmd.
Butter and margarine					
Light, 40% fat	1 tsp	0	0	2	Very Limited
	1 Tbsp	0	0	6	Very Limited
	2 Tbsp	0	0	11	Avoid
Regular	1 tsp	0	0	4	Very Limited
	1 pat	0	0	4	Avoid
	1 Tbsp	0	0	12	Avoid
	2 Tbsp	0	0	22	Avoid
	1 stick (½ cup)	0	0	92	Avoid

Food	Portion	Total Carbs (g)	Total Sugar (g)	Total Fat (g)	Recmmd.
Whipped butter, light	1 tsp	0	0	1	Very Limited
	1 Tbsp	0	0	4	Very Limited
	2 Tbsp	0	0	7	Avoid
Whipped butter, regular	1 tsp	0	0	3	Very Limited
	1 Tbsp	0	0	8	Avoid
	½ cup	0	0	60	Avoid
Butters, other					
Clarified butter (ghee)	1 Tbsp	0	0	14	Avoid
	2 Tbsp	0	0	28	Avoid
Garlic butter	1 Tbsp	0	0	11	Very Limited
Sweet cream butter, stick	1 Tbsp	0	0	10	Avoid
Sweet cream butter, tub	1 Tbsp	0	0	9	Avoid
Lard and animal fat					
Bacon grease	1 tsp	0	0	5	Avoid
Light and reduced-fat spreads					
Benecol-type, light spread	1 Tbsp	0	0	5	Good
Benecol-type, regular spread	1 Tbsp	0	0	9	Good

FATS (CONT.)

Food	Portion	Total Carbs (g)	Total Sugar (g)	Total Fat (g)	Recmmd.
Light and reduced-fat spreads (cont.)					
Butter substitutes, butter buds or sprinkles	1 Tbsp	0	0	1	Good
Cooking spray	2–3 second spray	0	0	1	Good
Country Crock–type, light	1 Tbsp	0	0	5	Very Limited
Country Crock–type, regular	1 Tbsp	0	0	7	Avoid
I Can't Believe It's Not Butter!–type, light	1 Tbsp	0	0	6	Very Limited
I Can't Believe It's Not Butter!–type, regular	1 Tbsp	0	0	10	Avoid
Parkay-type, squeeze bottle	1 Tbsp	0	0	9	Avoid
Parkay-type, stick or tub, ⅓ less fat	1 Tbsp	0	0	7	Avoid
Parkay-type, tub, light, soft	1 Tbsp	0	0	6	Very Limited
Weight Watchers–type, light	1 Tbsp	2	0	4	Very Limited

Food	Portion	Total Carbs (g)	Total Sugar (g)	Total Fat (g)	Recmmd.
Mayonnaise					
Dairy-free (soy-based, eggless)	1 Tbsp	1	0	4	Good
Fat-free	1 Tbsp	3	0	0	Avoid
Light	1 Tbsp	1	0	5	Limited
Regular	1 Tbsp	0	0	11	Limited
Miracle Whip–type salad dressing					
Fat-free	1 Tbsp	2	2	0	Limited
Light	1 Tbsp	2	2	3	Limited
Regular	1 Tbsp	2	1	7	Limited
Other fats					
Avocado	2 Tbsp	2	0	4	Good
Coconut, shredded, unsweetened	2 Tbsp	1	0	5	Limited
Coconut milk, canned, unsweetened	1 Tbsp	0	0	4	Limited
Olives, green, stuffed	10 large	0	0	5	Good
Olives, ripe, black	8 large	2	1	5	Good

FATS (CONT.)

Food	Portion	Total Carbs (g)	Total Sugar (g)	Total Fat (g)	Recmmd.
Vegetable shortening					
Vegetable shortening, conventional-type	1 Tbsp	0	0	13	Avoid
	2 Tbsp	0	0	28	Avoid
	1 cup	0	0	205	Avoid

OILS

Food	Portion	Total Carbs (g)	Total Sugar (g)	Total Fat (g)	Recmmd.
Avocado	1 Tbsp	0	0	14	Good
Canola	1 Tbsp	0	0	14	Good
Coconut	1 Tbsp	0	0	14	Limited
Corn	1 Tbsp	0	0	14	Limited
Cottonseed	1 Tbsp	0	0	14	Limited
Grapeseed	1 Tbsp	0	0	14	Limited
Olive	1 Tbsp	0	0	14	Good
Olive, extra virgin	1 Tbsp	0	0	14	Good
Palm	1 Tbsp	0	0	14	Limited
Palm kernel	1 Tbsp	0	0	14	Limited
Peanut	1 Tbsp	0	0	14	Good
Safflower	1 Tbsp	0	0	14	Limited
Sesame	1 Tbsp	0	0	14	Limited

Food	Portion	Total Carbs (g)	Total Sugar (g)	Total Fat (g)	Recmmd.
Soybean	1 Tbsp	0	0	14	Limited
Sunflower	1 Tbsp	0	0	14	Limited
Walnut	1 Tbsp	0	0	14	Good

FISH AND SHELLFISH

All fish is low in saturated fat, and many varieties of fish contain a good type of fat called omega-3. Omega-3, found in fish oil, appears to benefit us in several ways. As well as helping prevent heart attacks and strokes, there is evidence that fish oil helps prevent or treat depression, arthritis, colitis, asthma, and dry skin. It may also help us lose weight.

Shellfish, such as shrimp, were once labeled high in cholesterol, and avoided by people with concerns about their diets. But this has been proven wrong. Feel free to enjoy all shellfish on the South Beach Diet. However, the mercury content of fish is a growing concern. Canned tuna and swordfish should be limited for this reason.

FISH, BAKED OR BROILED

Food	Portion	Total Carbs (g)	Total Sugar (g)	Total Fat (g)	Recmmd.
Bass, sea	3 oz	0	0	2	Good
Bass, striped	3 oz	0	0	3	Good
Bluefish	3 oz	0	0	5	Good
Carp	3 oz	0	0	6	Good
Catfish	3 oz	0	0	9	Good
Cod	3 oz	0	0	1	Good
Flounder	3 oz	0	0	1	Good

FISH, BAKED OR BROILED (CONT.)

Food	Portion	Total Carbs (g)	Total Sugar (g)	Total Fat (g)	Recmmd.
Grouper	3 oz	0	0	1	Good
Haddock	3 oz	0	0	1	Good
Halibut	3 oz	0	0	2	Good
Herring	3 oz	0	0	10	Good
Herring, kippered, smoked	3 oz	0	0	10	Good
Lingcod, greenling	3 oz	0	0	1	Good
Mackerel	3 oz	0	0	15	Good
Mahi mahi	3 oz	0	0	1	Good
Monkfish	3 oz	0	0	2	Good
Ocean perch	3 oz	0	0	2	Good
Orange roughy	3 oz	0	0	1	Good
Pike	3 oz	0	0	1	Good
Pompano, Florida	3 oz	0	0	10	Good
Salmon					
King, chinook	3 oz	0	0	11	Good
Pink, chum	3 oz	0	0	4	Good
Red, sockeye	3 oz	0	0	9	Good
Smoked (lox)	3 oz	0	0	4	Good
Shark	3 oz	0	0	5	Good
Smelt, rainbow	3 oz	0	0	3	Good
Snapper	3 oz	0	0	2	Good
Sole	3 oz	0	0	1	Good
Sturgeon	3 oz	0	0	4	Good

Food	Portion	Total Carbs (g)	Total Sugar (g)	Total Fat (g)	Recmmd.
Swordfish	3 oz	0	0	4	Good
Trout, rainbow	3 oz	0	0	6	Good
Trout, sea	3 oz	0	0	4	Good
Tuna, fresh	3 oz	0	0	1	Good
Turbot	3 oz	0	0	3	Good
Whitefish, smoked	3 oz	0	0	6	Good
Whiting	3 oz	0	0	3	Good
Yellowtail	3 oz	0	0	6	Good

FISH, BREADED

Food	Portion	Total Carbs (g)	Total Sugar (g)	Total Fat (g)	Recmmd.
Clams, fried	3 oz	10	2	10	Avoid
Fish fillet, frozen, oven baked	3 oz	16	2	10	Avoid
Fish sticks, frozen, oven baked	3 oz	19	2	11	Avoid
Oysters, fried	3 oz	10	1	11	Avoid
Scallops, fried	3 oz	10	1	10	Avoid
Shrimp, fried	3 oz	19	2	10	Avoid

FISH, CANNED

Food	Portion	Total Carbs (g)	Total Sugar (g)	Total Fat (g)	Recmmd.
Anchovies, in oil, drained	3 oz	0	0	8	Good

FISH, CANNED (CONT.)

Food	Portion	Total Carbs (g)	Total Sugar (g)	Total Fat (g)	Recmmd.
Salmon, pink, drained	3 oz	0	0	4	Good
Sardines					
In mustard sauce, drained	3 oz	0	0	10	Good
In oil, drained	3 oz	0	0	10	Good
In tomato sauce, drained	3 oz	0	0	10	Good
In water, skinless	3 oz	0	0	9	Good
Tuna					
Light, in oil, drained	3 oz	0	0	7	Good
Light, in water, drained	3 oz	0	0	1	Good
White, in oil, drained	3 oz	0	0	7	Good
White, in water, drained	3 oz	0	0	1	Good

SHELLFISH, COOKED

Food	Portion	Total Carbs (g)	Total Sugar (g)	Total Fat (g)	Recmmd.
Clams	1 dozen (3 oz)	0	0	1	Good
Crab					
Blue, soft-shell	3 oz	0	0	1	Good
Dungeness	3 oz	0	0	1	Good
King, leg	3 oz	0	0	1	Good

Food	Portion	Total Carbs (g)	Total Sugar (g)	Total Fat (g)	Recmmd.
Crayfish	3 oz	0	0	1	Good
Lobster	3 oz	0	0	1	Good
Mussels	3 oz	0	0	2	Good
Oysters	6 medium (3 oz)	0	0	2	Good
Scallops	3 oz	0	0	1	Good
Shrimp	3 oz	0	0	2	Good

FRUIT AND FRUIT JUICES

Because of their carbohydrate, fiber, vitamin, and mineral content, most fruits can be eaten frequently after Phase 1. There are some that are high in sugar and should be eaten in limited amounts. We encourage the consumption of whole fruit. Avoid canned fruits packed in heavy syrup and processed commercial fruit juices.

FRUIT, CANNED

Food	Portion	Total Carbs (g)	Total Sugar (g)	Total Fat (g)	Recmmd.
Apricots, in light syrup	½ cup	19	17	0	Very Limited
Fruit cocktail, in natural juices	½ cup	14	13	0	Very Limited
Peaches					
In heavy syrup	½ cup	24	23	0	Avoid
In light syrup	½ cup	18	17	0	Very Limited
In natural juices	½ cup	14	13	0	Very Limited
Pear halves, in light syrup	½ cup	19	14	0	Very Limited

FRUIT, CANNED (CONT.)

Food	Portion	Total Carbs (g)	Total Sugar (g)	Total Fat (g)	Recmmd.
Pear halves, in natural juices	½ cup	21	17	0	Very Limited

FRUIT, DRIED

Food	Portion	Total Carbs (g)	Total Sugar (g)	Total Fat (g)	Recmmd.
Apples	1 oz	19	16	0	Good
Apricots	1 oz	24	20	0	Good
Currants	1 oz	21	19	0	Avoid
Dates, pitted	1 oz	21	18	0	Avoid
Figs	1 oz	37	30	0	Avoid
Prunes, pitted	1 oz	18	12	0	Good
Raisins	1 oz	22	18	0	Very Limited

FRUIT, FRESH

Food	Portion	Total Carbs (g)	Total Sugar (g)	Total Fat (g)	Recmmd.
Apple	1 small (4 oz)	16	12	0	Good
Applesauce, unsweetened	½ cup	15	12	0	Limited
Apricots	3 small (5 oz)	15	12	0	Good
Banana, ripe	1 small (3½ oz)	23	19	0	Limited
Blueberries	¾ cup	15	12	0	Good
Cantaloupe, melon	1 cup	13	12	0	Limited
Cherries, sour, pitted	1 cup	19	13	0	Good

Food	Portion	Total Carbs (g)	Total Sugar (g)	Total Fat (g)	Recmmd.
Cherries, sweet, pitted	1 cup	22	19	0	Limited
Cranberries	½ cup	6	4	0	Good
Grapefruit	½ large	16	10	0	Good
Grapes, red or green	1 cup (3¼ oz, 20 grapes)	16	15	0	Good
Kiwi	1 med. (3 oz)	12	8	0	Good
Lemon	1 med. (3 oz)	5	1	0	Good
Lime	1 med. (3 oz)	7	0	0	Good
Mango	1 small (3½ oz)	17	15	0	Limited
Nectarine	1 small (5 oz)	16	12	0	Good
Orange	1 small (6 oz)	19	15	0	Good
Papaya	1 small (8 oz)	22	13	0	Limited
Peach	1 med. (4 oz)	13	9	0	Good
Pear	1 med. (4 oz)	17	12	0	Good
Pineapple	1 cup	20	18	0	Very Limited
Plum	2 small (5 oz)	20	10	0	Good
Raspberries	1 cup	15	6	0	Good
Strawberries	1 cup	15	10	0	Good
Tangerine	1 med. (4 oz)	15	12	0	Good
Watermelon	1 cup	11	10	0	Avoid

FRUIT JUICES, UNSWEETENED

Food	Portion	Total Carbs (g)	Total Sugar (g)	Total Fat (g)	Recmmd.
Apple cider	½ cup	15	13	0	Limited

FRUIT JUICES, UNSWEETENED (CONT.)

Food	Portion	Total Carbs (g)	Total Sugar (g)	Total Fat (g)	Recmmd.
Apple juice	½ cup	15	13	0	Limited
Apricot nectar	½ cup	18	17	0	Very Limited
Banana juice	½ cup	10	10	0	Limited
Grape juice	½ cup	19	19	0	Limited
Grapefruit juice	½ cup	12	11	0	Limited
Mango nectar	½ cup	19	18	0	Very Limited
Orange juice, fresh	½ cup	13	12	0	Limited
Orange juice, reconstituted from frozen concentrate	½ cup	14	13	0	Very Limited
Papaya nectar	½ cup	18	15	0	Very Limited
Peach nectar	½ cup	17	16	0	Limited
Pear nectar	½ cup	19	18	0	Limited
Pineapple juice	½ cup	15	12	0	Very Limited
Prune juice	½ cup	23	17	0	Limited

GRAINS AND RICE

Enjoy grains frequently, as long as you eat the right ones. The more intact the grain, the higher the fiber and nutrition. Whole grains, including wheat, rye, barley, corn, and some types of rice, are rich in bran, B vitamins, iron, and other minerals. Stay away from white rice, which is milled, removing the bran and germ. Brown rice is a much better source of B vitamins, minerals, and fiber. Wild rice is frequently served in combination with white or brown rice and is very nutritious and low on the glycemic index. Couscous is another good low glycemic index choice to substitute for white rice or white potatoes.

GRAINS, COOKED

Food	Portion	Total Carbs (g)	Total Sugar (g)	Total Fat (g)	Recmmd.
Amaranth	½ cup	32	1	3	Avoid
Barley, pearled	½ cup	22	1	0	Good
Buckwheat (kasha)	½ cup	17	1	1	Good
Bulgur	½ cup	17	0	0	Good
Corn grits	½ cup	12	0	1	Limited
Cornmeal	½ cup	27	0	1	Limited
Couscous	½ cup	18	0	0	Limited
Millet	½ cup	21	0	1	Avoid
Oats, whole kernel	½ cup	26	1	3	Good
Rye, whole kernel	½ cup	29	2	1	Good
Wheat, whole kernel	½ cup	32	0	1	Good

RICE, COOKED

Food	Portion	Total Carbs (g)	Total Sugar (g)	Total Fat (g)	Recmmd.
Arborio risotto	½ cup	24	0	0	Limited
Basmati	½ cup	23	0	0	Limited
Brown	½ cup	23	0	1	Good
Brown, quick-cooking	½ cup	23	0	1	Avoid
Glutinous	½ cup	20	0	0	Avoid
Jasmine	½ cup	22	0	0	Avoid
White, instant	½ cup	20	0	0	Avoid
White, long-grain	½ cup	22	0	0	Limited
White, long-grain, converted-type	½ cup	22	0	0	Good
Wild	½ cup	18	1	0	Good

GRAVIES AND SAUCES

Canned or prepackaged gravies and sauces are often very high in sodium and fat, so read the labels carefully. When serving meat, stick to the natural, de-fatted meat juices.

GRAVIES

Food	Portion	Total Carbs (g)	Total Sugar (g)	Total Fat (g)	Recmmd.
Au jus	¼ cup	1	0	0	Good
Beef, mushroom, or turkey, canned	¼ cup	3	0	2	Very Limited
Beef, turkey, or chicken, fat-free, canned	¼ cup	3	1	0	Very Limited

Food	Portion	Total Carbs (g)	Total Sugar (g)	Total Fat (g)	Recmmd.
Chicken, canned	¼ cup	3	0	3	Very Limited
Homemade, thick	¼ cup	18	4	4	Very Limited
Mix, brown, prepared w/water	¼ cup	3	0	0	Very Limited

SAUCES

Food	Portion	Total Carbs (g)	Total Sugar (g)	Total Fat (g)	Recmmd.
Alfredo	¼ cup	5	2	18	Avoid
Béarnaise	¼ cup	5	2	19	Avoid
Béchamel (white sauce), thin, homemade	¼ cup	5	2	7	Very Limited
Bordelaise	¼ cup	5	1	6	Very Limited
Cheese fondue, homemade	¼ cup	2	0	7	Very Limited
Clam, red	¼ cup	6	3	1	Good
Clam, white	¼ cup	6	1	6	Limited
Hollandaise	¼ cup	5	1	18	Avoid
Marinara	¼ cup	8	5	1	Good
Mornay	¼ cup	6	3	15	Avoid
Peanut	¼ cup	7	2	11	Good
Pizza, unsweetened	¼ cup	7	2	0	Good

ICE CREAM AND FROZEN DESSERTS

Ice cream is not a part of the South Beach Diet, although you can enjoy a small amout as a *very* occasional treat. Opt for sugar-free fudge or fruit pops instead.

ICE CREAM

Food	Portion	Total Carbs (g)	Total Sugar (g)	Total Fat (g)	Recmmd.
Low-fat					
Neapolitan, no sugar added	½ cup	13	4	3	Very Limited
Vanilla, 50% less fat	½ cup	15	15	3	Very Limited
Premium					
Butter pecan	½ cup	20	19	23	Avoid
Cookies and cream	½ cup	29	24	18	Avoid
French vanilla, 20% fat	½ cup	21	21	18	Avoid
Macadamia nut	½ cup	20	18	24	Avoid
Mint chocolate chip	½ cup	25	22	20	Avoid
Regular					
Chocolate	½ cup	19	18	7	Very Limited
Peach	½ cup	17	16	6	Very Limited
Strawberry	½ cup	18	18	6	Very Limited
Vanilla	½ cup	17	12	7	Very Limited

ICE CREAM BARS AND POPS

Food	Portion	Total Carbs (g)	Total Sugar (g)	Total Fat (g)	Recmmd.
Fudge pop, no sugar added	1 each	9	2	0	Good
Ice cream sandwich	1 each	22	15	6	Very Limited
Juice bar, fruit-juice sweetened	1 each	15	15	0	Limited
Klondike-type bar	1 each	24	19	19	Avoid
Nutty Buddy–type cone	1 each	22	17	14	Avoid
Popsicle-type, sugar-free	1 each	3	0	0	Good

FROZEN DESSERTS

Food	Portion	Total Carbs (g)	Total Sugar (g)	Total Fat (g)	Recmmd.
Frozen yogurt					
Chocolate, fat-free	½ cup	22	20	0	Very Limited
Chocolate, low-fat	½ cup	21	17	2	Very Limited
Chocolate, regular	½ cup	23	18	3	Very Limited
Vanilla or fruit, low-fat	½ cup	18	18	1	Very Limited
Vanilla or fruit, regular	½ cup	22	17	3	Very Limited
Ice milk, vanilla, chocolate, or strawberry	½ cup	15	15	3	Very Limited

FROZEN DESSERTS (CONT.)

Food	Portion	Total Carbs (g)	Total Sugar (g)	Total Fat (g)	Recmmd.
Snow cone, w/syrup, flavored	6 oz cone	64	64	0	Avoid
Tofu-based frozen dessert	½ cup	20	13	13	Avoid

MEATS, PROCESSED MEATS, AND MEAT SUBSTITUTES

Many beef options are appropriate for a heart-healthy diet. To select the leanest cuts, look for "round" or "loin" in the name.

Processed meats are those products which are made from meat, such as beef, chicken, or turkey, and then "processed" into a "form." These include bologna, bratwurst, hot dogs, jerky, and sausage. Most of these products contain sodium nitrate as a preservative for longer shelf life and are, as a rule, extremely high in saturated fat and sodium.

Tofu, tempeh, and other soy-based foods are all good meat substitutes. When you eat these, you also benefit from soy's cholesterol-lowering properties.

BEEF

Food	Portion	Total Carbs (g)	Total Sugar (g)	Total Fat (g)	Recmmd.
Beef roasts, lean					
Bottom round, braised	3 oz	0	0	6	Good
Eye round, roasted	3 oz	0	0	4	Good
Pot roast, arm, braised	3 oz	0	0	7	Good
Pot roast, blade, braised	3 oz	0	0	11	Limited
Rib eye, roasted	3 oz	0	0	11	Limited

Food	Portion	Total Carbs (g)	Total Sugar (g)	Total Fat (g)	Recmmd.
Shank, cross-cut, braised	3 oz	0	0	5	Good
Short ribs, braised	3 oz	0	0	15	Avoid
Sirloin tip, roasted	3 oz	0	0	6	Good
Beef steaks, lean					
London broil, flank	3 oz	0	0	9	Good
Porterhouse, broiled	3 oz	0	0	9	Good
Rib eye, broiled	3 oz	0	0	10	Limited
Sirloin strip, broiled	3 oz	0	0	7	Good
T-bone, broiled	3 oz	0	0	8	Good
Tenderloin, broiled	3 oz	0	0	8	Good
Top round, panfried	3 oz	0	0	4	Avoid
Top sirloin, broiled	3 oz	0	0	6	Good
Briskets					
Corned beef, braised	3 oz	0	0	16	Avoid
Flat half, braised	3 oz	0	0	8	Avoid
Point half, braised	3 oz	0	0	13	Avoid
Whole, braised	3 oz	0	0	9	Limited

BEEF (CONT.)

Food	Portion	Total Carbs (g)	Total Sugar (g)	Total Fat (g)	Recmmd.
Cubes, stew, or kebabs, braised or grilled	3 oz	0	0	10	Limited
Ground beef					
Extra-lean, baked or broiled	3 oz	0	0	13	Good
Lean, baked or broiled	3 oz	0	0	15	Limited
Regular, baked or broiled	3 oz	0	0	18	Limited

LAMB, LEAN

Food	Portion	Total Carbs (g)	Total Sugar (g)	Total Fat (g)	Recmmd.
Cubes, stew, or kebabs, braised or grilled	3 oz	0	0	7	Good
Leg of lamb					
Shank half, roasted	3 oz	0	0	6	Good
Sirloin half, roasted	3 oz	0	0	8	Good
Whole, roasted	3 oz	0	0	7	Good
Loin chop, broiled	3 oz	0	0	8	Good
Rib, roast, crown rack of lamb, roasted	3 oz	0	0	11	Limited
Rib chop, broiled	3 oz	0	0	8	Limited

PORK

Food	Portion	Total Carbs (g)	Total Sugar (g)	Total Fat (g)	Recmmd.
Pork chitterlings	1 oz	0	0	8	Avoid
Pork chops, lean					
Blade, braised	3 oz	0	0	11	Limited
Center loin, broiled	3 oz	0	0	7	Good
Sirloin, braised	3 oz	0	0	6	Good
Top loin, broiled	3 oz	0	0	5	Good
Pork cutlets, lean					
Center slice, smoked ham, broiled or panfried	3 oz	0	0	9	Limited
Cutlet, braised or panfried	3 oz	0	0	8	Limited
Sirloin roast cutlet, braised or panfried	3 oz	0	0	8	Good
Pork roasts, lean					
Boston blade, braised	3 oz	0	0	11	Limited
Center loin, roasted	3 oz	0	0	8	Good
Center rib, roasted	3 oz	0	0	9	Good
Fresh ham, whole, roasted	3 oz	0	0	6	Good
Half shank, roasted	3 oz	0	0	6	Good

PORK (CONT.)

Food	Portion	Total Carbs (g)	Total Sugar (g)	Total Fat (g)	Recmmd.
Pork roasts, lean (cont.)					
Sirloin, roasted	3 oz	0	0	7	Good
Tenderloin, roasted	3 oz	0	0	4	Good
Top loin, roasted	3 oz	0	0	6	Good
Ribs					
Back ribs, full-fat, roasted	3 oz	0	0	25	Avoid
Spareribs, country-style, lean, braised	3 oz	0	0	12	Avoid
Spareribs, full-fat, braised	3 oz	0	0	25	Avoid

PORK, CURED

Food	Portion	Total Carbs (g)	Total Sugar (g)	Total Fat (g)	Recmmd.
Bacon					
Bacon bits	1 Tbsp	0	0	1	Avoid
Breakfast strips, broiled	2 med. strips (½ ounce)	0	0	5	Avoid
Canadian, grilled	3 oz	0	0	4	Good
Ham, cured, roasted					
Boneless, extra-lean	3 oz	0	0	5	Good
Boneless, lean	3 oz	0	0	8	Good

Food	Portion	Total Carbs (g)	Total Sugar (g)	Total Fat (g)	Recmmd.
Canned, extra-lean	3 oz	0	0	4	Good
Canned, lean	3 oz	0	0	7	Good

VEAL, LEAN

Food	Portion	Total Carbs (g)	Total Sugar (g)	Total Fat (g)	Recmmd.
Cutlet, braised	3 oz	0	0	8	Good
Ground, broiled	3 oz	0	0	6	Good
Loin chop, braised	3 oz	0	0	8	Good
Shank, stewed	3 oz	0	0	4	Good

PROCESSED MEATS

Food	Portion	Total Carbs (g)	Total Sugar (g)	Total Fat (g)	Recmmd.
Hot dogs, cooked					
Beef, fat-free	1 each	0	0	0	Very Limited
Beef, light, reduced-fat	1 each	0	0	8	Avoid
Beef, regular	1 each	0	0	13	Avoid
Beef and pork	1 each	0	0	13	Avoid
Chicken	1 each	0	0	9	Avoid
Turkey and cheese	1 each	0	0	13	Avoid
Turkey and pork	1 each	0	0	13	Avoid

PROCESSED MEATS (CONT.)

Food	Portion	Total Carbs (g)	Total Sugar (g)	Total Fat (g)	Recmmd.
Sandwich meats					
Bologna, beef	2 oz	0	0	12	Avoid
Bologna, beef and pork	2 oz	0	0	16	Avoid
Bologna, chicken	2 oz	0	0	13	Avoid
Bologna, lebanon	2 oz	0	0	7	Avoid
Bologna, pork	2 oz	0	0	11	Avoid
Bologna, turkey	2 oz	0	0	9	Avoid
Chicken roll	2 oz	0	0	4	Limited
Corned beef	2 oz	0	0	4	Limited
Dried beef	2 oz	0	0	2	Limited
Ham, boiled, deli thin	2 oz	0	0	2	Good
Ham, chopped	2 oz	0	0	8	Good
Ham, honey loaf	2 oz	0	0	4	Very Limited
Ham, turkey	2 oz	0	0	1	Good
Pastrami, beef	2 oz	0	0	17	Avoid
Pastrami, turkey	2 oz	0	0	4	Good
Pickle and pimiento loaf	2 oz	0	0	12	Avoid
Salami, beef	2 oz	0	0	13	Avoid
Salami, genoa	2 oz	0	0	18	Avoid
Salami, hard	2 oz	0	0	17	Avoid
Turkey breast, smoked	2 oz	0	0	1	Good
Turkey roll	2 oz	0	0	4	Good

Food	Portion	Total Carbs (g)	Total Sugar (g)	Total Fat (g)	Recmmd.
Sausages, cooked					
Bratwurst	2 oz	0	0	14	Avoid
Italian, sweet	2 oz	0	0	15	Avoid
Kielbasa	2 oz	0	0	15	Avoid
Knockwurst	2 oz	0	0	19	Avoid
Pork, patty	2 oz	0	0	16	Avoid
Summer	2 oz	0	0	13	Avoid
Turkey, patty	2 oz	0	0	6	Limited

MEAT SUBSTITUTES

Food	Portion	Total Carbs (g)	Total Sugar (g)	Total Fat (g)	Recmmd.
Burgers and hot dogs					
Black bean burger	1 each	15	0	0	Good
Hot dog, Tofu Pup, frozen	1 each	28	0	3	Good
Seitan (wheat gluten), refrigerated, ready to serve	4 oz	4	0	0	Good
Tempeh soy burger	1 each	11	0	4	Good
Veggie burger	1 each	18	0	3	Good
Tempeh (soybean)					
Fakin' Bacon, tempeh strips	2 med. strips (1 oz)	0	0	2	Good
Five grain	⅓ package	15	0	4	Good

MEAT SUBSTITUTES (CONT.)

Food	Portion	Total Carbs (g)	Total Sugar (g)	Total Fat (g)	Recmmd.
Tempeh (soybean) (cont.)					
Original, plain	⅓ package	10	0	6	Good
Wild rice	⅓ package	13	0	5	Good
Tofu (soybean)					
Baked and seasoned, refrigerated, ready to serve	3 oz	6	0	5	Good
Raw, firm, refrigerated	3 oz	2	0	4	Good
Silken, refrigerated	3 oz	2	0	2	Good

MILK, MILK PRODUCTS, AND MILK SUBSTITUTES

Dairy products are an excellent source of calcium and protein and make for great snacks. But whole-milk dairy products, such as butter, cheese, milk, cream, and ice cream contain high amounts of saturated fat. When selecting dairy products, look for non-fat or low-fat varieties of milk or plain yogurt or yogurt sweetened with aspartame. These products contain the milk sugar lactose, which has a moderated glycemic index lower than other simple sugars. Also look for low-fat soy milk and soy drinks, which contain more protein and less fat than cow's milk.

CREAMS AND CREAMERS

Food	Portion	Total Carbs (g)	Total Sugar (g)	Total Fat (g)	Recmmd.
Cream					
Half & half	2 Tbsp	1	0	3	Very Limited

Food	Portion	Total Carbs (g)	Total Sugar (g)	Total Fat (g)	Recmmd.
Light	2 Tbsp	1	0	6	Limited
Medium	2 Tbsp	1	0	7	Very Limited
Creamers, nondairy					
Liquid, refrigerated, fat-free	2 Tbsp	4	0	0	Good
Liquid, refrigerated, flavored, sweetened	2 Tbsp	10	10	4	Avoid
Liquid, refrigerated, light	2 Tbsp	2	0	2	Good
Liquid, refrigerated, regular, plain	2 Tbsp	4	2	4	Limited
Powdered, original	1 tsp	1	1	2	Good
Sour cream					
Fat-free	2 Tbsp	3	2	0	Good
Imitation, plain	2 Tbsp	2	2	5	Limited
Nondairy, substitute, plain	2 Tbsp	1	0	5	Limited
Reduced-fat	2 Tbsp	2	2	3	Good
Regular, plain	2 Tbsp	1	1	5	Limited

CREAMS AND CREAMERS (CONT.)

Food	Portion	Total Carbs (g)	Total Sugar (g)	Total Fat (g)	Recmmd.
Toppings, whipped					
Dessert cream topping, frozen, extra-creamy	2 Tbsp	2	2	2	Very Limited
Dessert cream topping, frozen, light	2 Tbsp	2	1	1	Good
Dessert cream topping, frozen, nondairy	2 Tbsp	2	1	2	Good
Whipped cream, pressurized	2 Tbsp	1	1	2	Very Limited
Whipping cream					
Heavy, liquid	1 Tbsp	1	1	6	Avoid
Heavy, whipped	¼ cup	1	1	11	Avoid
Heavy, whipped, from ½ cup liquid	1 cup	3	3	44	Avoid
Light, liquid	1 Tbsp	1	1	5	Avoid
Light, whipped	¼ cup	1	1	9	Avoid
Light, whipped, from ½ cup liquid	1 cup	4	4	37	Avoid

MILK AND NONDAIRY MILKS

Food	Portion	Total Carbs (g)	Total Sugar (g)	Total Fat (g)	Recmmd.
Buttermilk, low-fat, 1%	8 fl oz	12	12	3	Good

Food	Portion	Total Carbs (g)	Total Sugar (g)	Total Fat (g)	Recmmd.
Buttermilk, reduced-fat, 2%	8 fl oz	12	12	5	Limited
Chocolate Milk					
Low-fat, 1%	8 fl oz	26	22	3	Very Limited
Reduced-fat, 2%	8 fl oz	26	22	5	Avoid
Whole milk	8 fl oz	26	22	8	Avoid
Cow's milk					
Fat-free/skim	8 fl oz	12	12	0	Good
Low-fat/light, 1%	8 fl oz	12	12	3	Good
Protein-fortified	8 fl oz	14	14	5	Limited
Reduced-fat, 2%	8 fl oz	12	12	5	Very Limited
Whole, 3.5%	8 fl oz	12	12	8	Avoid
Eggnog, reduced-fat	4 fl oz	17	17	8	Very Limited
Eggnog, regular	4 fl oz	17	17	10	Avoid
Low-lactose					
Fat-free	8 fl oz	12	12	0	Good
Low-fat, 1%	8 fl oz	12	12	3	Good
Reduced-fat, 2%	8 fl oz	12	12	5	Avoid
Other milks and kefir					
Acidophilus milk, low-fat, 1%	8 fl oz	12	12	3	Good
Acidophilus milk, reduced-fat, 2%	8 fl oz	12	12	5	Limited

MILK AND NONDAIRY MILKS (CONT.)

Food	Portion	Total Carbs (g)	Total Sugar (g)	Total Fat (g)	Recmmd.
Other milks and kefir (cont.)					
Goat's milk, low-fat	8 fl oz	9	9	3	Good
Goat's milk, whole	8 fl oz	11	11	10	Avoid
Kefir, plain	8 fl oz	11	11	8	Avoid
Canned milk					
Evaporated, fat-free	2 Tbsp	4	4	0	Good
Evaporated, low-fat	2 Tbsp	3	3	1	Good
Evaporated, whole	2 Tbsp	3	3	2	Avoid
Sweetened condensed, fat-free	2 Tbsp	24	24	0	Avoid
Sweetened condensed, low-fat	2 Tbsp	23	23	2	Avoid
Sweetened condensed, regular	2 Tbsp	21	21	3	Avoid
Dry milk					
Buttermilk	1 oz	14	14	2	Good
Nonfat	1 oz	15	15	0	Good
Whole milk	1 oz	12	12	8	Avoid

Food	Portion	Total Carbs (g)	Total Sugar (g)	Total Fat (g)	Recmmd.
SOY MILK					

Food	Portion	Total Carbs (g)	Total Sugar (g)	Total Fat (g)	Recmmd.
Chocolate, refrigerated	8 fl oz	23	19	4	Limited
Plain, refrigerated	8 fl oz	8	4	4	Good
Soy milk creamer, refrigerated	2 Tbsp	2	0	2	Good
Unsweetened, refrigerated	8 fl oz	5	1	4	Good
Vanilla, refrigerated	8 fl oz	10	7	4	Limited

YOGURTS

Food	Portion	Total Carbs (g)	Total Sugar (g)	Total Fat (g)	Recmmd.
Fruited					
Fat-free, sweetened w/sugar	8 oz	39	31	0	Avoid
Light, fat-free, artificially sweetened	8 oz	22	17	0	Limited
Low-fat, drinkable	8 oz	36	34	3	Very Limited
Low-fat, sweetened w/sugar	8 oz	43	37	2	Avoid
Whole milk, sweetened w/sugar	8 oz	38	31	6	Avoid

YOGURTS (CONT.)

Food	Portion	Total Carbs (g)	Total Sugar (g)	Total Fat (g)	Recmmd.
Plain					
Fat-free	8 oz	18	12	0	Good
Low-fat	8 oz	16	16	4	Limited
Whole milk	8 oz	11	11	7	Avoid
Soy yogurt, fruited, sweetened w/evaporated cane juice	8 oz	38	28	3	Avoid
Soy yogurt, plain	8 oz	22	12	3	Good

NUTS, NUT BUTTERS, AND SEEDS

News of the positive health benefits of nuts continues to accumulate. Nuts are a great source of good fats and protein, and consumption of nuts has been associated with decreased risks of heart attacks. Almonds, Brazil nuts, peanuts, pistachios, and many other nuts are all good choices. Natural nut butters appear to have the same health benefits as whole nuts, but it is important to read the labels to make sure that hydrogenated oils are not listed as ingredients. Smuckers, for example, has a natural peanut butter made without trans fats that is a good choice.

NUTS

Food	Portion	Total Carbs (g)	Total Sugar (g)	Total Fat (g)	Recmmd.
Almonds, raw or roasted	1 oz	7	2	14	Good
Brazil nuts, raw	1 oz	4	1	19	Good
Cashews, roasted	1 oz	10	2	14	Good

Food	Portion	Total Carbs (g)	Total Sugar (g)	Total Fat (g)	Recmmd.
Filberts (hazelnuts), roasted	1 oz	5	1	17	Good
Macadamias, raw	1 oz	5	2	20	Good
Peanuts, roasted	1 oz	6	1	14	Good
Pecans, dried	1 oz	5	1	19	Good
Pine nuts, dried	1 oz	6	1	15	Good
Pistachios, shelled	1 oz	8	2	13	Good
Soy nuts, roasted	1 oz	9	2	6	Good
Walnuts, English, dried	1 oz	5	1	18	Good

NUT BUTTERS

Food	Portion	Total Carbs (g)	Total Sugar (g)	Total Fat (g)	Recmmd.
Almond butter	1 Tbsp	3	2	9	Good
Cashew butter	1 Tbsp	5	1	7	Good
Hazelnut butter	1 Tbsp	3	2	10	Good
Peanut butter, reduced-fat	1 Tbsp	8	2	6	Good
Peanut butter, w/no added sugar, freshly ground	1 Tbsp	4	1	8	Good
Pistachio butter	1 Tbsp	5	2	9	Good
Sesame seed paste (tahini)	1 Tbsp	2	0	9	Good
Soy nut butter	1 Tbsp	6	1	6	Good

SEEDS

Food	Portion	Total Carbs (g)	Total Sugar (g)	Total Fat (g)	Recmmd.
Flaxseed	1 Tbsp	3	0	3	Good
Poppy	1 Tbsp	2	0	3	Good
Pumpkin (pepitas)	1 Tbsp	2	0	4	Good
Sesame	1 Tbsp	2	0	4	Good
Sunflower	1 Tbsp	2	0	4	Good

PASTA AND PASTA DISHES

Whole wheat pasta is the preferred type of pasta on the South Beach Diet. We recommended that you boil the pasta until just tender or "al dente." Also, to reduce portion size, try eating pasta as a side dish to your fish or chicken, rather than a stand-alone entrée.

Enjoy your pasta with a low-sugar tomato sauce. Research shows that lycopene in tomatoes can be more efficiently absorbed when processed into tomato sauces or tomato paste. This is important because lycopene has been shown to help prevent prostate cancer.

PASTA, COOKED

Food	Portion	Total Carbs (g)	Total Sugar (g)	Total Fat (g)	Recmmd.
Capellini, semolina	1 cup	43	2	1	Very Limited
Corn pasta, gluten-free	1 cup	39	3	1	Avoid
Egg noodle, homemade, plain, spinach, or tomato	1 cup	40	2	2	Very Limited
Fettuccine, egg noodle, spinach	1 cup	40	2	2	Very Limited

Food	Portion	Total Carbs (g)	Total Sugar (g)	Total Fat (g)	Recmmd.
Linguine, semolina	1 cup	42	1	1	Very Limited
Macaroni, semolina	1 cup	39	2	1	Very Limited
Macaroni, whole wheat	1 cup	38	1	1	Limited
Rice pasta, brown	1 cup	39	1	2	Limited
Spaghetti, semolina	1 cup	41	1	1	Very Limited
Spaghetti, whole wheat	1 cup	39	1	1	Limited
Vermicelli, semolina	1 cup	42	2	1	Very Limited

PASTA DISHES, PREPARED WITH SEMOLINA PASTA

Food	Portion	Total Carbs (g)	Total Sugar (g)	Total Fat (g)	Recmmd.
Gnocchi, potato dumpling	1 cup	75	11	3	Avoid
Lasagna, w/meat sauce, homemade	1 cup	38	6	16	Very Limited
Lasagna, w/spinach, vegetarian, homemade	1 cup	41	7	10	Very Limited
Macaroni and cheese, baked, homemade	1 cup	30	6	12	Avoid
Macaroni and cheese, prepared from box	1 cup	49	8	18	Avoid

PASTA DISHES, PREPARED WITH SEMOLINA PASTA (CONT.)

Food	Portion	Total Carbs (g)	Total Sugar (g)	Total Fat (g)	Recmmd.
Meat ravioli, w/meat sauce	1 cup	36	7	17	Avoid
Meat ravioli, w/tomato sauce	1 cup	38	10	14	Avoid
Pasta primavera	1 cup	47	4	11	Avoid
Spaghetti					
W/marinara sauce	1 cup	42	12	5	Very Limited
W/meatballs and marinara sauce	1 cup	36	6	12	Avoid
W/red clam sauce	1 cup	41	8	8	Very Limited
W/white clam sauce	1 cup	43	5	20	Avoid
Tortellini, cheese, w/tomato sauce	1 cup	43	2	10	Avoid

PICKLES, PEPPERS, AND RELISH

Pickles, peppers, and relishes are all okay as long as they are not the sweetened versions.

Food	Portion	Total Carbs (g)	Total Sugar (g)	Total Fat (g)	Recmmd.
Bread and butter pickles, sweetened	3 pieces	5	5	0	Avoid
Dill pickle	1 large	5	2	0	Limited

Food	Portion	Total Carbs (g)	Total Sugar (g)	Total Fat (g)	Recmmd.
Gherkin, sweet	1 medium	5	5	0	Very Limited
Green chiles, chopped	2 Tbsp	2	1	0	Good
Jalapeño peppers, pickled	2 whole	2	0	0	Limited
Peppers, roasted, whole, red or yellow, jarred	½ of whole	2	1	2	Good
Sauerkraut, drained	½ cup	3	0	0	Good
Sweet gherkin pickle relish, sweetened	1 Tbsp	5	5	0	Avoid

PIZZA

If pizza is among your favorite treats, have a thin-crust pizza with tomato sauce, reduced-fat cheese, and/or vegetables. Thick-crust pizzas, as well as those made on French bread, are trouble. Also steer clear of high saturated fat toppings, such as mixed cheeses, pepperoni, and sausage.

FRENCH BREAD PIZZA, FROZEN

Food	Portion	Total Carbs (g)	Total Sugar (g)	Total Fat (g)	Recmmd.
Deluxe cheese	1 serving	45	2	19	Avoid
Pepperoni	1 serving	47	3	20	Avoid
Sausage	1 serving	48	5	21	Avoid
White cheese	1 serving	45	2	23	Avoid

PIZZA, TRADITIONAL

Food	Portion	Total Carbs (g)	Total Sugar (g)	Total Fat (g)	Recmmd.
Personal Pan Pizza					
Beef	10 oz slice	71	2	35	Avoid
Cheese	9¼ oz slice	71	3	28	Avoid
Ham	9 oz slice	70	2	23	Avoid
Italian sausage	10¼ oz slice	71	2	39	Avoid
Pepperoni	9 oz slice	70	2	28	Avoid
Pork	9 oz slice	71	2	34	Avoid
12" Hand-Tossed Pizza					
Cheese	3½ oz slice	43	8	10	Avoid
Pepperoni	3½ oz slice	43	8	13	Avoid
Sausage	4 oz slice	44	8	14	Avoid
Vegetable	4½ oz slice	45	9	6	Avoid
12" Pan Pizza					
Cheese	4 oz slice	44	2	13	Avoid
Pepperoni	4½ oz slice	44	2	14	Avoid
Sausage	4½ oz slice	45	2	18	Avoid
Vegetable	4½ oz slice	46	2	12	Avoid
12" Thin Crust Pizza					
Cheese	3 oz slice	28	1	8	Good
Pepperoni	3 oz slice	29	1	10	Avoid
Sausage	3½ oz slice	29	1	12	Avoid

Food	Portion	Total Carbs (g)	Total Sugar (g)	Total Fat (g)	Recmmd.
Whole Wheat Pizza, frozen					
Four cheese	2¾ oz slice	19	2	7	Good
Mushroom and spinach	2¾ oz slice	21	3	4	Good
Vegetarian	2¾ oz slice	17	3	4	Good

POULTRY

When it comes to chicken, bake, broil, grill, roast, or sauté, but do not fry.

Select the chicken breast, which has far less saturated fat than the leg, thigh, and wing, and remove the skin before eating. Duck and goose are higher in saturated fat than chicken and should not be eaten often.

CHICKEN (AN AVERAGE OF LIGHT AND DARK MEAT)

Food	Portion	Total Carbs (g)	Total Sugar (g)	Total Fat (g)	Recmmd.
Fried, batter-dipped	4 oz	11	0	20	Avoid
Fried, flour-coated	4 oz	5	0	17	Avoid
Roasted, w/skin	4 oz	0	0	15	Very Limited
Roasted, without skin	4 oz	0	0	8	Good
Stewed, w/skin	4 oz	0	0	14	Very Limited
Stewed, without skin	4 oz	0	0	8	Good

CHICKEN, ORGAN MEATS, SIMMERED

Food	Portion	Total Carbs (g)	Total Sugar (g)	Total Fat (g)	Recmmd.
Giblets	½ cup	1	0	4	Avoid
Gizzard	½ cup	1	0	3	Very Limited
Heart	½ cup	1	0	6	Avoid
Liver	½ cup	1	0	4	Avoid

CHICKEN, PARTS, BROILERS OR FRYERS

Food	Portion	Total Carbs (g)	Total Sugar (g)	Total Fat (g)	Recmmd.
Breast (½ breast)					
Fried, batter-dipped, w/skin	5 oz	12	0	19	Avoid
Fried, flour-coated, w/skin	3½ oz	7	0	9	Avoid
Roasted, w/skin (from 5 oz raw)	3½ oz	0	0	8	Very Limited
Roasted, without skin (from 4¼ oz raw)	3 oz	0	0	3	Good
Stewed, w/skin	3½ oz	0	0	8	Very Limited
Stewed, without skin	3 oz	0	0	3	Good
Drumstick					
Fried, batter-dipped, w/skin	2½ oz	6	0	10	Avoid
Fried, flour-coated, w/skin	1¾ oz	4	0	7	Avoid
Roasted, w/skin	2 oz	0	0	6	Very Limited

Food	Portion	Total Carbs (g)	Total Sugar (g)	Total Fat (g)	Recmmd.
Roasted, without skin	1½ oz	0	0	2	Limited
Stewed, w/skin	2 oz	0	0	6	Very Limited
Stewed, without skin	1½ oz	0	0	3	Limited
Thigh					
Fried, batter-dipped, w/skin	3 oz	8	0	14	Avoid
Fried, flour-coated, w/skin	2¼ oz	5	0	9	Avoid
Roasted, w/skin (from 4 oz raw w/bone)	2½ oz	0	0	10	Very Limited
Roasted, without skin (from 4 oz raw w/bone)	2 oz	0	0	6	Limited
Stewed, w/skin	2½ oz	0	0	10	Very Limited
Stewed, without skin	2 oz	0	0	5	Limited
Wing					
Fried, batter-dipped, w/skin	1¾ oz	5	0	11	Avoid
Fried, flour-coated, w/skin	1 oz	1	0	7	Avoid
Roasted, w/skin (from 3 oz raw w/bone)	1¼ oz	0	0	7	Very Limited
Roasted, without skin (from 2½ raw w/bone)	¾ oz	0	0	2	Good

CHICKEN, ROASTERS

Food	Portion	Total Carbs (g)	Total Sugar (g)	Total Fat (g)	Recmmd.
Dark meat, without skin, roasted	3 oz	0	0	9	Limited
Light and dark meat (an average), roasted w/skin	4 oz	0	0	15	Very Limited
Light and dark meat (an average), roasted without skin	4 oz	0	0	8	Limited
Light meat, without skin, roasted	3 oz	0	0	4	Good

CHICKEN, STEWING

Food	Portion	Total Carbs (g)	Total Sugar (g)	Total Fat (g)	Recmmd.
Dark meat, without skin	3 oz	0	0	16	Limited
Light and dark meat, (an average), w/skin	4 oz	0	0	21	Very Limited
Light and dark meat, (an average), without skin	4 oz	0	0	14	Limited
Light meat, without skin	3 oz	0	0	9	Good

TURKEY

Food	Portion	Total Carbs (g)	Total Sugar (g)	Total Fat (g)	Recmmd.
Dark meat, w/skin	3½ oz	0	0	7	Very Limited
Dark meat, without skin	3 oz	0	0	4	Limited
Light meat, w/skin	3½ oz	0	0	5	Limited
Light meat, without skin	3 oz	0	0	1	Good
Turkey parts					
Back, roasted, w/skin	4½ oz	0	0	12	Very Limited
Back, roasted, without skin	3½ oz	0	0	5	Limited
Breast meat, roasted, w/skin,	4¼ oz	0	0	10	Very Limited
Breast meat, roasted, without skin	3 oz	0	0	2	Good
Giblets, simmered	1 cup	0	0	7	Avoid
Leg (thigh and drumstick), roasted, w/skin	8¼ oz	0	0	13	Very Limited
Leg (thigh and drumstick), roasted, without skin	7½ oz	0	0	8	Limited
Neck, simmered, w/bone	9 oz	0	0	11	Very Limited
Wing, roasted, w/skin	3 oz	0	0	9	Very Limited

TURKEY (CONT.)

Food	Portion	Total Carbs (g)	Total Sugar (g)	Total Fat (g)	Recmmd.
Turkey parts (cont.)					
Wing, roasted, without skin	2 oz	0	0	2	Good

CAPON, CORNISH HEN, DUCK, AND GOOSE

Food	Portion	Total Carbs (g)	Total Sugar (g)	Total Fat (g)	Recmmd.
Capon, roasted, ½ chicken, w/skin	23 oz	0	0	74	Very Limited
Capon, roasted, w/skin	4 oz	0	0	13	Very Limited
Cornish hen, roasted					
Dark meat, w/skin	3 oz	0	0	11	Very Limited
Dark meat, without skin	3 oz	0	0	7	Limited
Light meat, w/skin	3 oz	0	0	8	Very Limited
Light meat, without skin	3 oz	0	0	3	Good
Duck, roasted, w/skin	3 oz	0	0	24	Very Limited
Duck, roasted, without skin	3 oz	0	0	10	Very Limited
Goose, roasted, w/skin	3 oz	0	0	19	Very Limited
Goose, roasted, without skin	3 oz	0	0	11	Very Limited

SALADS AND SALAD DRESSINGS

Prepared salads, such as tuna or egg, can be an occasional part of your diet, but the best salads are those with mixed greens and a flavorful vinaigrette dressing.

SALADS

Food	Portion	Total Carbs (g)	Total Sugar (g)	Total Fat (g)	Recmmd.
Antipasto	1 cup	5	1	10	Limited
Bean salad	1 cup	23	6	5	Good
Caesar salad, w/dressing	1 cup	15	2	15	Good
Chef salad, w/turkey, ham, and cheese, no dressing	1 cup	7	3	11	Limited
Chicken salad spread	½ cup	9	4	19	Avoid
Coleslaw, traditional, sweetened	½ cup	18	13	9	Very Limited
Cucumber salad, marinated in vinaigrette	½ cup	8	5	10	Good
Egg salad	½ cup	8	1	25	Very Limited
Fresh fruit salad	1 cup	25	22	0	Limited
Greek pasta salad, w/olives and feta cheese	1 cup	42	8	12	Limited
Grilled chicken salad	½ cup	13	9	10	Good
Macaroni salad, traditional, w/egg	1 cup	42	13	23	Avoid

SALADS (CONT.)

Food	Portion	Total Carbs (g)	Total Sugar (g)	Total Fat (g)	Recmmd.
Pasta salad, w/Italian vinaigrette	1 cup	42	5	12	Very Limited
Potato salad, traditional, w/egg	1 cup	38	7	19	Avoid
Shrimp salad	½ cup	5	2	14	Good
Tabbouleh salad	½ cup	22	1	6	Good
Tomato salad, w/mozzarella	1 cup	20	12	14	Good
Tortellini salad, w/pesto	1 cup	38	6	20	Avoid
Tossed green salad	1 cup	10	0	0	Good
Tuna salad, traditional, w/egg	½ cup	10	4	12	Good
Waldorf salad	1 cup	24	12	21	Avoid

SALAD DRESSINGS

Food	Portion	Total Carbs (g)	Total Sugar (g)	Total Fat (g)	Recmmd.
Blue cheese, reduced-fat	2 Tbsp	2	1	8	Good
Blue cheese, regular	2 Tbsp	2	2	16	Limited
Caesar, reduced-fat	2 Tbsp	1	0	5	Good
Caesar, regular	2 Tbsp	2	0	14	Good
French					
Fat/oil-free	2 Tbsp	4	2	0	Very Limited

Food	Portion	Total Carbs (g)	Total Sugar (g)	Total Fat (g)	Recmmd.
Reduced-fat	2 Tbsp	7	6	3	Very Limited
Regular	2 Tbsp	5	5	14	Avoid
Italian					
Fat/oil-free	2 Tbsp	2	1	0	Good
Reduced-fat	2 Tbsp	2	2	7	Good
Regular	2 Tbsp	3	3	12	Good
Ranch					
Fat-free	2 Tbsp	2	1	0	Good
Reduced-fat	2 Tbsp	3	1	8	Good
Regular	2 Tbsp	3	3	18	Limited
Russian					
Fat-free	2 Tbsp	2	1	0	Limited
Reduced-fat	2 Tbsp	2	2	5	Limited
Regular	2 Tbsp	3	3	10	Very Limited
Thousand Island					
Fat-free	2 Tbsp	3	1	0	Limited
Reduced-fat	2 Tbsp	3	3	4	Limited
Regular	2 Tbsp	5	4	11	Very Limited
Vinaigrette, balsamic, fat-free	2 Tbsp	8	8	0	Avoid
Vinaigrette, balsamic, regular	2 Tbsp	3	3	10	Good

SOUPS

A first course of soup will not only soothe your spirits, it will satisfy your appetite. Research shows that people given a first course of tomato soup ate less during subsequent courses. Good choices also include vegetable soups, such as bean, gazpacho, and lentil, which are all packed with good carbs and fiber.

Avoid cream-type soups in restaurants because they are usually made with saturated fat-laden heavy cream or whole milk. At home, make cream-type soups with water. When ordering French onion soup you might want to order it without the French bread topping.

Food	Portion	Total Carbs (g)	Total Sugar (g)	Total Fat (g)	Recmmd.
Barley mushroom	1 cup	19	4	1	Good
Beef barley	1 cup	20	2	2	Good
Beef vegetable	1 cup	17	3	2	Good
Black bean	1 cup	19	2	2	Good
Bouillabaisse	1 cup	6	2	9	Good
Chicken noodle	1 cup	18	1	2	Very Limited
Chicken rice	1 cup	17	1	2	Very Limited
Clam chowder					
Manhattan, red	1 cup	20	3	4	Very Limited
New England, reduced-fat	1 cup	18	1	3	Very Limited
New England, white	1 cup	20	3	10	Very Limited
Corn chowder, creamy	1 cup	18	4	15	Avoid

Food	Portion	Total Carbs (g)	Total Sugar (g)	Total Fat (g)	Recmmd.
Cream soups					
Cream of broccoli, made w/water	1 cup	17	5	3	Good
Cream of chicken, made w/water	1 cup	18	4	4	Good
Cream of mushroom, made w/milk	1 cup	15	6	13	Avoid
Cream of potato, made w/milk	1 cup	16	2	9	Avoid
French onion soup	1 cup	22	10	4	Limited
Fish chowder	1 cup	18	5	6	Good
Gazpacho	1 cup	4	2	0	Good
Lentil	1 cup	22	2	1	Good
Lentil w/ham	1 cup	20	2	3	Good
Lobster bisque	1 cup	13	10	13	Avoid
Minestrone	1 cup	20	3	3	Good
Miso broth	1 cup	5	0	0	Good
Split pea	1 cup	30	2	2	Limited
Tomato	1 cup	15	8	2	Good
Vegetable	1 cup	15	3	1	Good
Vegetable, w/turkey	1 cup	14	3	4	Good
Vichyssoise	1 cup	17	2	6	Limited

SWEETENERS AND SWEET SUBSTITUTES

Naturally occurring sugars are those found in foods like milk products (lactose) and fruits (fructose). Refined sugars include honey, maple syrup, and table sugar. Most sugars have a low to moderate ranking on the glycemic index. Table sugar (sucrose) has a moderate ranking and can be included as part of an occasional treat or as an ingredient in baking.

However, sugar is the number one additive to our food supply. The typical person eats approximately 32 teaspoons of added sugar a day. Some high fructose corn syrup will be added even to products using sugar substitutes. Read and compare labels and choose wisely.

CANE SUGAR

Food	Portion	Total Carbs (g)	Total Sugar (g)	Total Fat (g)	Recmmd.
Brown sugar	1 tsp	13	13	0	Very Limited
Raw sugar, turbinado	1 tsp	12	12	0	Very Limited
White sugar, granulated	1 tsp	4	4	0	Very Limited
	1 Tbsp	12	12	0	Avoid
	¼ cup	50	48	0	Avoid
	½ cup	100	98	0	Avoid

JAMS, JELLIES, AND FRUIT SPREADS

Food	Portion	Total Carbs (g)	Total Sugar (g)	Total Fat (g)	Recmmd.
Fruit butter, apple	1 Tbsp	8	6	0	Avoid
Fruit spreads, 100% fruit	1 Tbsp	11	8	0	Avoid
Jam or jelly, light	1 Tbsp	9	7	0	Avoid
Jam or jelly, regular	1 Tbsp	14	10	0	Avoid

Food	Portion	Total Carbs (g)	Total Sugar (g)	Total Fat (g)	Recmmd.
Marmalade, orange	1 Tbsp	13	12	0	Avoid
Preserves, reduced-sugar	1 Tbsp	9	7	0	Avoid
Preserves, regular	1 Tbsp	13	12	0	Avoid

OTHER SUGARS

Food	Portion	Total Carbs (g)	Total Sugar (g)	Total Fat (g)	Recmmd.
Fructose	10 grams	10	10	0	Good
Glucose	10 grams	10	10	0	Avoid
Lactose	10 grams	10	10	0	Good
Maltose	10 grams	10	10	0	Avoid
Sucrose	10 grams	10	10	0	Limited

SUGAR SUBSTITUTES

Food	Portion	Total Carbs (g)	Total Sugar (g)	Total Fat (g)	Recmmd.
Equal (aspartame)	1 tsp	0	0	0	Allowed
Splenda (sucralose)	1 tsp	0	0	0	Allowed
Sprinkle Sweet (saccharin)	1 tsp	0	0	0	Allowed
Stevia	1 tsp	0	0	0	Not FDA Approved
Sugar Twin (saccharin)	1 tsp	0	0	0	Allowed
Sweet'N Low (saccharin)	1 tsp	0	0	0	Allowed

SUGAR SUBSTITUTES (CONT.)

Food	Portion	Total Carbs (g)	Total Sugar (g)	Total Fat (g)	Recmmd.
Sweet One (acesulfame K)	1 tsp	0	0	0	Allowed
Sweet-Ten (saccharin)	1 tsp	0	0	0	Allowed

SYRUPS

Food	Portion	Total Carbs (g)	Total Sugar (g)	Total Fat (g)	Recmmd.
Corn syrup, high-fructose	1 tsp	14	14	0	Avoid
Honey, commercial blend	1 tsp	17	17	0	Avoid
Honey, pure	1 tsp	17	17	0	Very Limited
Maple syrup, pure	1 tsp	13	13	0	Very Limited
Pancake syrup, imitation, maple	1 tsp	14	9	0	Avoid
Pancake syrup, imitation, reduced-calorie	1 tsp	7	6	0	Avoid

VEGETABLES

Eat and enjoy plenty of vegetables. They are low in calories but high in vitamins, essential nutrients, and fiber. Look for brightly colored vegetables, which contain antioxidants, such as Vitamins A, C, and E. Opt for as much variety as possible, and yes, even carrots are fine. In addition to their nutrient contribution, vegetables, especially when eaten raw, are a great source of fiber and bulk. When cooked in water, vegetables quickly lose their nutrients, so when you cook your vegetables do so in as little water as possible, and for as short a time as possible.

Food	Portion	Total Carbs (g)	Total Sugar (g)	Total Fat (g)	Recmmd.
Artichokes	½ cup	8	1	0	Good
Asparagus	½ cup	4	1	0	Good
Beans, green	½ cup	4	2	0	Good
Beets	½ cup	8	6	0	Limited
Bok choy	½ cup	2	0	0	Good
Broad beans (fava)	½ cup	8	1	0	Limited
Broccoli	½ cup	4	2	0	Good
Broccoli rabe	½ cup	3	1	0	Good
Brussels sprouts	½ cup	7	3	0	Good
Cabbage, green or red	½ cup	3	1	0	Good
Carrots	½ cup	8	5	0	Good
Cauliflower	½ cup	3	1	0	Good
Celery	½ cup	3	1	0	Good
Chicory, raw	1 cup	4	0	0	Good
Chives, raw	2 Tbsp	0	0	0	Good
Cilantro, raw	2 Tbsp	0	0	0	Good
Collards	½ cup	5	0	0	Good
Corn, sweet	½ cup	18	2	1	Very Limited
Cucumber, raw	½ cup	1	0	0	Good
Daikon radish, white	½ cup	3	1	0	Good
Dandelion greens, raw	1 cup	5	1	0	Good

VEGETABLES (CONT.)

Food	Portion	Total Carbs (g)	Total Sugar (g)	Total Fat (g)	Recmmd.
Eggplant	½ cup	3	2	0	Good
Endive, raw	1 cup	4	0	0	Good
Fennel	½ cup	3	0	0	Good
Garlic	1 clove	0	0	0	Good
Ginger, juice or grated	1 tsp	0	0	0	Good
Green onion (scallion), raw	2 Tbsp	0	0	0	Good
Kale	½ cup	3	1	0	Good
Kohlrabi	½ cup	6	4	0	Good
Leeks	½ cup	4	1	0	Good
Lettuce, raw	1 cup	2	0	0	Good
Mushrooms	½ cup	4	0	0	Good
Mustard greens	½ cup	1	0	0	Good
Okra	½ cup	4	1	0	Good
Onions	½ cup	9	7	0	Good
Parsley, raw	2 Tbsp	0	0	0	Good
Parsnips	½ cup	15	4	0	Very Limited
Peas					
Green	½ cup	16	4	0	Limited
Snow, pod	½ cup	5	3	0	Good
Sugar snap	½ cup	7	3	0	Good
Pepper, bell, red or green	½ cup	3	1	0	Good
Pepper, chile, raw	2 Tbsp	1	1	0	Good

Food	Portion	Total Carbs (g)	Total Sugar (g)	Total Fat (g)	Recmmd.
Potatoes, baked, w/skin					
Extra-large	12 oz	86	5	0	Avoid
Large	8 oz	57	4	0	Avoid
Medium	5 oz	36	2	0	Avoid
Small	3 oz	21	1	0	Avoid
Potatoes, other					
Instant mashed	½ cup	18	1	0	Avoid
Mashed, regular, plain, no fat	½ cup	18	1	0	Avoid
Microwaved, whole	5 oz	36	2	0	Avoid
New, whole	2½ oz	9	0	0	Limited
Pumpkin	½ cup	6	4	0	Very Limited
Purslane	½ cup	2	0	0	Good
Radish, red	½ cup	2	1	0	Good
Rutabaga	½ cup	7	3	0	Very Limited
Sauerkraut	½ cup	3	0	0	Good
Shallots	2 Tbsp	0	0	0	Good
Sorrel, raw	2 Tbsp	1	0	0	Good
Spinach, raw	1 cup	2	0	0	Good
Sprouts, alfalfa, raw	½ cup	0	0	0	Good
Squash, yellow summer	½ cup	3	1	0	Good

VEGETABLES (CONT.)

Food	Portion	Total Carbs (g)	Total Sugar (g)	Total Fat (g)	Recmmd.
Sweet potato, cubes, baked	½ cup	21	11	0	Good
Swiss chard	½ cup	4	0	0	Good
Tomato, ripe	1 cup	7	4	0	Good
Tomato juice, unsweetened	1 cup	11	7	0	Good
Tomatoes, cooked	½ cup	4	3	0	Good
Tomatillo, raw	1 cup	7	4	0	Good
Turnip	½ cup	4	2	0	Good
Watercress	½ cup	0	0	0	Good
Wax beans	½ cup	4	2	0	Good
Yam, cubes, baked	½ cup	19	1	0	Good
Zucchini	½ cup	2	1	0	Good

THE SOUTH BEACH SUPERMARKET CHEAT SHEET

There's nothing worse than arriving home from work hungry and discovering that the cupboard is bare. Keep the following staple items in your freezer and pantry, and you'll always have the makings of a healthy South Beach meal.

Dairy

Reduced-fat or fat-free cheese: Try American, Cheddar, mozzarella, ricotta, and Swiss—you'll find countless varieties. Experiment with different brands until you find one you like.

Fat-free plain yogurt: Use it as a staple for making "cream" sauces or dips. (Put it in a sieve lined with a coffee filter and refrigerate it for 3 or more hours, then combine it with your favorite seasonings.)

Flavor Boosters

Balsamic vinegar: It wakes up salads, is a fat-free way to sauté, and is great combined with olive oil in marinades.

Garlic: No well-stocked kitchen is complete without garlic, a staple of Mediterranean cuisine.

Olive and canola oils. For the best-tasting salad dressings, light sautéing, dips for bread, or dressing for steamed vegetables, buy extra virgin olive oil. Canola oil is good for stir-fries.

Onions: Keep a couple of these on hand: red, yellow, and white onions; shallots; and scallions.

Salsa: Use fresh or jarred salsa in place of ketchup and as an accompaniment for grilled meat, poultry, or seafood.

Sesame oil and reduced-sodium soy sauce: These flavor boosters add instant Asian flavor to steamed vegetables, stir-fries, and marinades. Refrigerating these items will help them preserve their flavor if you don't use them up quickly.

Meat, Poultry, and Fish

Boneless top sirloin: For quick and easy beef-and-vegetable kebabs, skewer the meat with mushrooms and chunks of red pepper and onion.

Boneless turkey and chicken breast: Grill it, bake it, or use it in stir-fries.

Veggies and Beans

Beans: Try all kinds—black, butter, lentils, limas, kidney, chickpeas, green, Italian, and split peas.

Frozen vegetables: Keep broccoli and cauliflower florets, asparagus, and chopped spinach on hand for stir-fries, sautéed or microwaved side dishes, additions to casseroles and soups, and Mediterranean dishes like ratatouille.

Prewashed, prepackaged broccoli florets: Serve them as no-fuss crudités with reduced-fat or fat-free cheese, sauté them with black beans as a side dish, or add them to a ready-made soup.

MEDLEY OF
MENU MAKEOVERS

It's one thing to follow a straight-from-the-book diet plan, quite another to assemble your own healthy meals. But it's not as hard as it may seem. Simply pair a serving of lean protein with a serving of fiber-rich, fresh veggies (other than high-glycemic varieties like corn and potatoes). Add a dash of healthy oils. Presto—you've got a delicious meal that slows your digestion and keeps you feeling satisfied for hours.

These before-and-after breakfast, lunch, and dinner "makeovers" will help inspire you to think of your own tempting combos. Pair what you know about the nutritional principles of the diet with your own favorite foods and a little creativity and the sky's the limit.

SWITCH FROM THIS . . .   **. . . TO THIS**

BREAKFAST

Omelet with cheese, hash browns, bacon or pork sausage, and orange juice (from concentrate)

Veggie omelet, Canadian bacon, an orange, and fat-free milk

Plain bagel and a mocha latte

One slice whole wheat toast with no sugar-added peanut butter and coffee with 1% milk and sugar substitute

Pancakes topped with syrup

Whole grain pancakes topped with fresh fruit

LUNCH

Salad with fat-free dressing and pasta with red sauce

Tossed salad with olive oil and vinegar dressing (vinaigrette) and whole grain pasta with shrimp and veggies

Cheeseburger and fries

Grilled chicken breast sandwich on a whole grain roll

Veggie wrap

Tuna salad and veggies wrapped in lettuce

DINNER

Fried chicken, white rice, and a biscuit

Baked chicken breast, steamed asparagus, and a tossed salad with vinaigrette

Meat loaf, mashed potatoes, and bread spread with margarine

Broiled sirloin steak, sweet potato, and oven-roasted veggies

Pork barbecue on a bun, corn, and a tossed salad with fat-free dressing

Cup of tomato soup, open-faced roast beef sandwich, and a tossed salad with vinaigrette

THE SOUTH BEACH
DINING-OUT GUIDE

You don't have to stop frequenting your favorite restaurants just because you're on the South Beach Diet. This way of eating is flexible so that you can find several healthy choices that allow you to enjoy the dining-out experience and still lose or maintain weight. This cheat sheet will help you select the healthiest choices virtually anywhere—even at ethnic restaurants.

Regardless of which Phase of the Diet you're on, be guided by the ground rules for South Beach eating.

Chain Restaurants

Upscale chains offer so much variety that there's plenty to choose from other than deep-fried appetizers, huge entrée portions, and frozen margaritas. At all chain restaurants, avoid appetizers smothered in cheese and sour cream (such as nachos or potato skins), sandwiches called melts (tuna melt, for instance, which are loaded with cheese and grilled with butter), croissant sandwiches, coleslaw, macaroni and potato salads, and fried tortilla shell or bread "bowls."

Try these instead:

At Boston Market: A quarter of a chicken, white meat, no skin or wing; a chicken, turkey, or ham sandwich without cheese or dressing; any fresh vegetable, such as green beans or broccoli.

At Chili's: The Guiltless Grill items, which are usually served with black beans or steamed veggies; shrimp, chicken, or beef fajitas, topped with salsa and minus the flour tortillas and full-fat cheese and sour cream.

At Ruby Tuesday: The salad bar, which contains all the makings for a healthy salad (greens, chickpeas, fresh vegetables, diced turkey or ham, olive oil and balsamic dressing); a turkey burger without the bun; grilled chicken or grilled-chicken salads without the cheese or deep-fried tortilla bowl.

Chinese Food

To give Americanized Chinese food a South Beach makeover, minimize the huge amounts of saturated fat used to prepare it. Ask that your dish be prepared without MSG, the flavoring agent often used in Chinese cuisine. While it's made from beets, a healthy vegetable, MSG has a very high glycemic index (GI). Try egg drop soup or any combination of steamed fresh vegetables prepared with small amounts of meat, poultry, or seafood. Stay away from: steamed rice (it has a high GI); the deep-fried, crispy noodles; egg rolls; fried dumplings; spareribs; lo mein; moo goo gai pan; Peking duck; and entrées described on the menu as "crispy" or "sweet and sour." Also, many sauces may be thickened with cornstarch. Ask the waiter for sauces prepared without added cornstarch.

Indian Food

Indian food is based on good carbs, particularly legumes like chickpeas and lentils, and veggies such as spinach and eggplant. The downside is its abundance of starchy carbs (like potatoes) and bad fats. Many appetizers are deep-fried, and vegetables and meats are typically fried or sautéed in the Indian butter called *ghee*. Still, most Indian restaurants provide several tasty choices for the South Beach dieter. Try Mulligatawny soup, dals (legume dishes—choose those without cream), chana (chickpea curry), kachumbars (vegetable salads), raitas (salads with a tart yogurt dressing), or dishes described on the menu as masala (a combination of spices with sautéed tomatoes and onions) or tandoori (seasoned meat, poultry, or fish roasted in a clay oven).

Stay away from Samosas (deep-fried pastry filled with vegetables or meat); puri (a puffy, deep-fried bread); and entrées described as biryani, malai, or korma, which are heavy on the oil and cream.

Italian Food

Not order pasta? At an Italian restaurant? Actually, it's easier than you think—there are usually several choices right for the South Beach dieter. Try salads dressed with oil and balsamic vinegar; clams steamed in white wine; clear soups; grilled meat, poultry, or fish; scallops sautéed with mushrooms and marsala wine sauce; or escarole or broccoli rabe (two types of greens) sautéed in garlic and olive oil.

If you order pizza, request a thin-crust pie rather than Sicilian or deep-dish, and pile it with veggies rather than sausage or pepperoni. If you must have pasta, ask for whole wheat pasta and order a side serving sautéed in olive oil and garlic or topped with plain tomato sauce and good proteins (clams or shrimp) or vegetables. Stay away from bread or garlic bread; antipastos with cheeses and salami, which are high in saturated fat; and anything described on the menu as "carbonara" (prepared with full-fat cream and cheese) or parmigiana (breaded, fried, and smothered in full-fat mozzarella).

Mexican Food

Most Mexican food at chain restaurants and Mexican fast-food places is prepared American-style, which means an abundance of bad fats. Yet it is possible to go Mexican and eat healthfully. Try grilled chicken or fish, *pescado Veracruzana* (fish in a tangy sauce of olive oil, grilled onions, green olives, and capers), *mole pollo* (boned chicken breast served in a hot and spicy sauce), *mojo pollo* (chicken in a tangy citrus sauce), or *camarones de hacha* (shrimp sautéed in a red and green tomato sauce). Stay away from deep-fried tortilla chips; anything topped with cheese, sour cream, or guacamole; refried beans (commonly fried in lard); chimichangas (deep-fried flour tortillas filled with meat and cheese); the Mexican sausage called chorizo; and deep-fried taco-shell bowls.

Steak Houses

You should be able to have a good South Beach meal in a restaurant specializing in steaks and vegetables. Order a lean cut of meat and enjoy it with a cup of broth-based soup and a side dish of steamed or grilled vegetables.

Try lean cuts of beef such as top sirloin or tenderloin or a well-trimmed lamb or pork loin chop (ask that the extra fat be trimmed away before cooking). At the salad bar, opt for peel-and-eat shrimp, shrimp cocktail, and salad greens with broccoli and other nonstarchy vegetables dressed with olive oil and balsamic vinegar.

Stay away from deep-fried appetizers, creamy soups such as New England clam chowder, baby back ribs, coleslaw, macaroni and potato salads, baked potatoes, steak fries, and onion rings.

INDEX

Underscored page references indicate charts.

NOTES

Since the diet became popular in Miami and the book *The South Beach Diet* became a bestseller, I've heard from countless people eager to tell me about their weight loss successes. I'm encouraged by how easy the program is to learn and put into practice. Now there is a Web site designed to make the diet even easier: www.southbeachdiet.com/rodale.

How? The Web site has the flexibility to provide personal feedback and guidance to help you reach your goals. It also has the ability to put you in touch with thousands of others following the plan. In the Message Boards, you'll be able to ask questions and get answers from a large community of dieters with similar experiences, as well as from our expert nutritionists. You'll get regular advice from me, too, in the Daily Dish newsletter and the Ask Dr. Agatston Q&As.

The site's interactive tools are also designed to provide personal support. In the Weight Tracker, for instance, you can key in your weight, chart your progress, and get immediate feedback on how you're doing on the diet. The site will tell you if you're losing weight too fast or too slow, and what you can do about it. It's like having your own personal trainer pointing out areas for improvement, telling you that you're doing better than you think, and keeping you motivated.

In the Meal Plans section of the site, you'll find Daily Menus for whatever phase of the diet you're in, a Recipe Search to help you find delicious new dishes quickly and easily (including vegetarian-only recipes), and a Shopping List Generator that will print out lists of ingredients automatically. By following the South Beach Diet Online, you'll not only get help gaining control of your weight and your heart health, you'll also be helping us make the diet better. Science is changing and improving all the time, and I see this diet as an evolution. As we learn new information about dieters' needs and experiences, we'll be able to continually improve the Web site, the plan, and our ability to help people. To learn about changes and updates to the diet without registering for this site, visit www.southbeachdiet.com/updates

Arthur Agatston, M.D.